PRACTICAL
ON NURSING PR...

PRACTICAL NOTES ON NURSING PROCEDURES

JESSIE D. BRITTEN S.R.N.
Sister Tutor Diploma (London), Trained at Royal Free Hospital, Formerly Registered Nurse Tutor, Worcester Royal Infirmary

FOREWORD BY

George H. Marshall F.R.C.S. (Edin.)
Consultant Surgeon to
Worcester Royal Infirmary

SIXTH EDITION

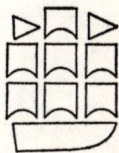

CHURCHILL LIVINGSTONE
EDINBURGH AND LONDON 1971

CHURCHILL LIVINGSTONE
Medical Division of Longman Group Limited

Distributed in the United States of America by Longman Inc., New York, and by associated companies, branches and representatives throughout the world.

© Longman Group Limited, 1974

All rights reserved. No part of this publication may be reproduced, stored in a retrieval system, or transmitted in any form or by any means, electronic, mechanical, photocopying, recording or otherwise, without the prior permission of the publishers (Churchill Livingstone, 23 Ravelston Terrace, Edinburgh).

First Edition	1957
Second Edition	1959
Third Edition	1960
Revised Reprint	1962
Fourth Edition	1963
Reprinted	1964
Fifth Edition	1966
Reprinted	1968
Sixth Edition	1971
Reprinted	1974
Second Reprint	1974

ISBN 0 443 00788 8

FOREWORD

The continuing popularity of this book makes me all the more proud that I have been asked to write a Foreword.

Seldom in the history of modern medicine have trained nurses been required to make so many alterations in time honoured procedures or student nurses been asked to adopt so many new procedures and it is with the help of an immediate reference book of this variety that they will be enabled to master and perform their practical duties.

We live in an age of new man-made fabrics and substances many of which have revolutionized surgical equipment and technique and also at a time when infection is better understood than ever before and methods of sterilisation even more efficient than we had thought could be achieved. These things indeed have improved our techniques making them all the more safe for the performance of medical and surgical work than at any time in the past. But reliance on them and shelter behind a shower of antibiotics cannot bring total success unless the person employing them also plays his, or her, individual and important part. It is no doubt with such things in mind that this book goes into its new edition so that the nurse can see in an easily understandable way how she is to perform practical duties and achieve best results. She is the essential link between inventors and manufacturers of improved equipment and the all important participant in the work, her patient. On her at all times there hangs a heavy burden of conscientious exactness in detail of day-to-day procedure for no matter how perfect may be the equipment or how potent may be the drug, its power and success still lie in the correctness of its use.

Worcester.   G. H. MARSHALL

PREFACE TO THE SIXTH EDITION

In revising this book, I have endeavoured to bring it up to date, by deleting many of the now obsolete practices, replacing them with modern methods. I hope, as a result, that it will continue to be of value to the Student and Pupil Nurse.

My very grateful and sincere thanks to Miss M. A. Priest, Principal Nursing Officer, (Teaching Division) of the United Bristol Hospitals Group, for the great work she did in helping me with the revision of this edition.

My renewed thanks go to E. & S. Livingstone, for the courtesy shown at all times and for the interest and hard work in the publication of this book.

1971　　　　　　　　　　　　　　　　　　　　J. D. BRITTEN

PREFACE TO THE FIRST EDITION

In compiling this book I have endeavoured to give a concise outline, enhanced with clear drawings of basic nursing procedures (using the General Nursing Council Syllabus as a guide), which I hope will be of value to Student Nurses and also to Pupil Nurses.

To Miss C. M. Turner, Principal Tutor, Worcester Royal Infirmary, I wish to extend my very grateful thanks, for without her ever-ready help and encouragement this book could not have been written.

My thanks are also due to Miss V. C. Whiter for reading the manuscript, and to all other persons who have in any way helped in collecting the material.

I am greatly indebted to Miss Elizabeth Hardman, Matron, Royal Free Hospital, for having read the proofs and written the foreword.

I wish also to extend my sincere thanks to Mr Charles Macmillan for his untiring help and encouragement. To Mr R. W. Matthews, who undertook the tremendous task of producing the illustrations with such excellent results, and to all other members of the staff of E. & S. Livingstone Ltd., who have helped in the preparation and publication of this book.

Lastly, I wish to thank Misses Ross and Wilson from whom the blocks for Figures 23 and 24 were borrowed.

1957   J. D. BRITTEN

CONTENTS

CHAPTER   PAGE

I. THE HOSPITAL AND THE NURSE 1
The hospital as a unit—Recent nursing history—Ethics—Legal aspects for nurses—Psychological aspects of nursing—Teaching of health.

II. THE WARD AND ANNEXES 19
General management—Cleaning and care of equipment—Economy.

III. BEDMAKING 26
Care of beds and bedding, linen—Routine and special bedmaking—Positions used—Bed accessories—Filling hot water bottles.

IV. GENERAL CARE OF PATIENT 47
Admission, discharge, last offices—Bed bathing—Bathing children and infants—Infant feeding—Prevention of bedsores—Care of mouth, teeth, hands, feet and hair——Giving and removing bedpans—Getting patient up—Care of the ambulant patient.

V. TEMPERATURE, PULSE AND RESPIRATION, BLOOD PRESSURE 67
Variations in health and disease—Rules for taking and recording.

VI. EXCRETA,—URINE TESTING, ENEMATA . . . 74
Observation and saving specimens of urine, faeces, sputum, vomit—Urine testing—Administration of fluids by rectum—Use of rectal tube—Fluid intake and output measurement.

VII. INFECTION AND DISINFECTION. WARD DRESSINGS . 88
Infection, sterilisation, disinfection—Central Sterile Supply Department—Ward dressing technique.

VIII. ADMINISTRATION OF MEDICINES 95
Weights and measures—Rules for administering medicines by mouth—Alternative routes—Hypodermic and intramuscular injections.

IX. INHALATIONS AND OXYGEN 103
Moist and dry inhalations—Methods of giving oxygen.

X. PREPARATION FOR OPERATION. GENERAL OBSERVATIONS 110
Preparation of patient for operation—Pre-operative shaving—Care and observation after general anaesthetic—General observation of patient—Care of the unconscious patient.

CONTENTS

CHAPTER		PAGE
XI.	PREPARATION OF PATIENT FOR VARIOUS EXAMINATIONS	117
	Physical—X-ray—Radium therapy—Endoscopy—Dilatation and curettage.	
XII.	LOCAL APPLICATIONS. BATHS	129
	Cold—Hot—Counter-irritants—Miscellaneous—Medicated baths—Sponging.	
XIII.	EXTENSIONS. PLASTER OF PARIS. SPLINTS	138
XIV.	CATHETERISATION	145
	Female and male.	
XV.	VARIETIES OF WASHOUT PROCEDURES	149
	Bladder washout and drainage—Rectal and colostomy washout—Vaginal douching—Insertion of pessaries—Stomach washout—Gastric aspiration.	
XVI.	EAR, NOSE AND THROAT TREATMENTS	162
	Syringing and swabbing ear—Instillation of drops—Cleaning nose, instillation of drops—Spraying and painting throat—Tracheotomy—Antrostomy—Myringotomy—Peritonsillar abscess—Control of nasal bleeding.	
XVII.	EYE TREATMENTS	170
	Instillation of drops—Swabbing, spoon bathing and irrigation.	
XVIII.	ARTIFICIAL FEEDING	173
	Gastrostomy—Jejunostomy—Oesophageal and nasal.	
XIX.	INFUSIONS	177
	Subcutaneous, intravenous and intramedullary—Blood donors.	
XX.	DRAINAGE AND EXPLORATION OF BODY CAVITIES	183
	Exploration and aspiration of chest—Artificial pneumothorax—Paracentesis abdominis—Southey's tubes—Lumbar puncture.	
XXI.	LABORATORY EXAMINATIONS	189
	Urine concentration, urea clearance and concentration tests—Blood tests—Cerebro-spinal fluid—Sternal puncture—Fractional test meal—Histamine test—Glucose tolerance test.	
XXII.	ANAESTHETICS. ARTIFICIAL RESPIRATORS	197
	Preparation for anaesthetics—Hypothermia—Types of respirators—Care of patient.	
	APPENDIX	202
	INDEX	209

Chapter One

THE HOSPITAL AND THE NURSE

The hospital as a unit—Recent nursing history—Ethics—Legal aspects for nurses—Psychological aspects of nursing—Teaching of health

THE HOSPITAL AS A UNIT

The main function of a hospital is to cater for the sick and injured with the object of:

1. Diagnosing disease or injury.
2. Curing disease or injury.
3. Alleviating suffering when cure is not possible.
4. Carrying on research into the causes of disease, and the means of curing and preventing it.

In order to accomplish this, the hospital is divided into many departments, each dealing with a particular part of the work. All these departments are inter-dependent, and the smooth, successful running of a hospital as a whole depends on the efficiency and co-operation of each department.

Hospitals are now run under tripartite administration *i.e.* three main areas:

1. Administration.
2. Nursing (*a*) Education.
   (*b*) Service.
3. Medicine.

These include the following departments:

1. General Administration. (Stores accounts, wages, records, clerical staff, porters, cleaners, residences, linen, transport.)
2. Nursing Administration. (Staff, tutoring.)
3. Social Services—Medical Social Workers.
4. Surgical.
5. Burns.
6. Plastic Surgery.
7. Cardiac and Chest Surgery.
8. Intensive Care.
9. Operating Theatres.
10. Recovery or Post-anaesthetic Wards.
11. Gynaecology.

12. Urology.
13. Artificial Kidney.
14. Orthopaedic.
15. Neuro-surgical.
16. Ear, Nose and Throat.
17. Eye.
18. Medical.
19. Psychiatric.
20. Paediatric.
21. X-ray, Diagnostic and Therapeutic.
22. Physiotherapy.
23. Occupational Therapy.
24. Rehabilitation Centre.
25. Laboratories. (Clinical, bacteriological, histological.)
26. Accident.
27. Out-Patients.
28. Pharmacy.
29. Geriatric.
30. Central Sterile Supply.

AN EXAMPLE OF HOSPITAL ROUTINE

A patient who has had an accident is taken to the Accident Department. If necessary, *i.e.* the patient is unconscious, the semi-prone position is adopted and immediate resuscitation carried out, *e.g.* patient's own heat conserved, or in some cases patient is kept cool. If conscious, nothing given by mouth if patient is likely to require an anaesthetic.

A doctor will endeavour to ascertain the extent of injury and order any appropriate treatment. It is important to record, in writing, name, dosage and time of any drugs given.

A nurse will obtain particulars about the patient from relatives or friends. It may be necessary to send patient to X-ray department, or if too ill a portable X-ray machine may be used. If he or she is in urgent need of an operation, *e.g.* cut throat, he or she may be prepared for operation, and sent directly to Operating Theatre from Accident department. Meanwhile, Theatre Sister and Ward Sister must be advised of this. Minor operations are carried out in Casualty Theatre. If the injuries do not require immediate operative treatment, but call for admission to a ward, arrangements must be made with the appropriate Ward Sister. A written report of all treatment given must accompany the patient to the ward.

Minor injuries attending Accident Department for the first time are often expected to go to a Records Office first, to give their particulars and receive a record card. After treatment, this card is entered up and returned to the Records Office, and the patient must call for it at each subsequent visit.

OUT-PATIENTS

These are patients who have either been sent to see a consultant by their own doctor, who will have made an appointment for them, or have been in-patients and have been told to return and see their particular consultant, at a specific time. In the first case, the home doctor will send a note with the patient, who will again have to give his particulars at the Record Office, and receive an Out-patient book. This book is returned to the office by the receptionist after the patient has been seen. It must be collected from the office on each subsequent visit by the patient, before he sees the consultant.

In-patients will have been issued with a small card bearing their index number, when they were discharged from the ward. On presenting this to the receptionist on their first visit to the Out-patient Department she will be able to obtain their in-patient notes; they may then be issued with an out-patient book.

Dentists attend Out-patient Departments only to deal with the jaws and mouth of patients referred to them by the consultant staff, as requiring special treatment prior to operation. They do not attend for the purpose of ordinary dentistry, which must be done by the patient's own dentist. If a person comes to hospital with extreme toothache, the doctor on casualty duty may remove the tooth.

Consultants order the necessary treatment. Resident doctors and sisters co-operate in seeing that it is carried out. The promptness and efficiency with which the orders are carried out plays a vital part in the successful treatment of the patient and in the smooth running of the hospital.

THE MINISTRY OF HEALTH AND SOCIAL SECURITY

All matters concerning the health of the people are in charge of a central authority, the Ministry of Health and Social Security.

The Minister of Health is in charge.

His advisers are:

1. The Chief Medical Officer of Health.
2. The Chief Nursing Officer.
3. Assistants, both professional, executive and clerical.

THE CENTRAL AUTHORITY prepares and supervises the implementation of Acts of Parliament dealing with health matters. Usually laws are administered in all parts of the country by Local

Authorities, either County Councils or County Borough Councils, but the National Health Service Act is an exception, because hospital services are administered by special machinery set up for the purpose under the Act, *i.e.* Regional Hospital Boards.

GENERAL PRACTITIONER SERVICES are administered by Executive Councils under the control of General Medical Councils.

PUBLIC HEALTH SERVICES are administered by the local Authorities.

THE NATIONAL HEALTH SERVICE is largely financed from taxation. THE NATIONAL HEALTH SERVICE ACT, 1946, provides for a Health Service organised in three main parts under the control of the Ministry of Health, namely:

1. Hospital and Consultant Services.
2. General Practitioner Services. Dentistry, Ophthalmology, Pharmacy.
3. Local Health Authority Services.

This set up is under review, as the three divisions of the N.H.S. tend not to communicate enough for satisfactory service to the public.

RECENT NURSING HISTORY DEVELOPMENT
The Nurses Act, 1949

In January 1949, a Working Party was organised resulting in the passing of the Nurses Act.

When the Health Services of the country became nationalised in 1948, it was decided by the Ministry of Health that the training of student nurses should be re-organised, and accordingly the Nurses Act was drawn up and received the Royal Assent on 24th November 1949, but was not implemented until 22nd September 1950.

Under the Act, certain moneys are set aside solely for the use of Nurse Training Schools, to enable experimental work to be carried out and so ultimately to arrive at the most suitable methods for the training of nurses. It was arranged for the establishment of Area Nurse Training Committees, and these have now been appointed for each of the fifteen regional areas for England and Wales.

These Committees are to advise and assist the training institutions in the regional hospital areas in all matters connected with the training of nurses; to advise and, if asked to do so, to assist the General Nursing Council in matters relating to the approval of training institutions, and to promote improvements and research into training methods. Each Committee consists of fifteen members representative of all types of hospitals in the region, and the greater majority of members are trained nurses.

Provision is also made in the Act for the persons who do not wish to take the three year training for State Registration. It is possible for them to take a two-year course and become State Enrolled Nurses.

The General Nursing Council

This Council is a statutory body working directly with the Department of Health and Social Security. It came into existence in 1919 after Nurses had struggled for more than thirty years for legal recognition of the status of the Nursing Profession. It was reorganised under the Nurses Act 1949 and the elections held throughout England and Wales enable State Registered Nurses to vote for seventeen registered nurses to form half of the General Nursing Council (the remaining seventeen being appointed by other bodies). These registered nurses (seventeen) are representative of the whole of the country, as prior to the elections the whole of England and Wales was divided up into fifteen regions so that the nurses themselves have been able to elect a truly representative section of the whole country. Of the seventeen State Registered Nurses, fourteen are general trained nurses, male and female; one must be a sick children's nurse; two must be mental nurses (one male and one female). The remaining seventeen members have been appointed as follows: three by the Minister of Education, two by the Privy Council (of whom one represents the Universities of England and Wales) and twelve have been appointed by the Minister; of the twelve, two are Registered Nurse Tutors; two Nurses employed in chronic nursing; one Registered Male Nurse; one Ward Sister and three persons with experience of the control and management of hospitals. Thus the newly constituted General Nursing Council is truly representative.

Briefly the work of the General Nursing Council will consist of:

1. EDUCATION AND EXAMINATIONS.—A Committee draws up the conditions of training (length, minimum requirements). Syllabus of subjects for examinations. Conditions relating to examinations and their conduct; has liaison with Universities regarding approval of Nurse Tutor Courses; gives approval of pre-nursing courses on the recommendation of the Ministry of Education.

2. A PSYCHIATRIC NURSING COMMITTEE.—Has the same function as above, but for the Psychiatric Nurse Training.

3. A REGISTRATION COMMITTEE.—Maintaining a register of all

State Registered Nurses and to give special consideration to those who trained in other countries before admitting them to the State Register. Maintaining a register of qualified Nurse Tutors and Clinical Instructors recognised by the General Nursing Council.

4. ENROLMENT COMMITTEE for maintaining roll of State Enrolled Nurses.

5. DISCIPLINARY AND PENAL CASES COMMITTEE.—Where State Registered Nurses are convicted of a felony or misdemeanour—names may be removed from the Register, being restored at a later date if the Committee considers it advisable. The Council also has the power to prosecute persons who falsely claim the title of Nurse.

6. FINANCE COMMITTEE.—Deals with all monetary matters of the General Nursing Council, and allocates available money for the running of Nurse Training Schools.

The above notes are only a very brief summary of the work of the General Nursing Council, but it is the watchdog of the profession, constantly on guard to see that the level of the training does not fall below a certain minimum so that State Registration guarantees a high standard of efficiency.

To simplify the organisation of Nurse Training, an index of students was commenced in June 1947; every Candidate who enters for training must be registered with the General Nursing Council within thirty days of entering the Preliminary Training School. She is given a number which she carries with her throughout her training, using it in any correspondence she has with the General Nursing Council.

With the introduction of this index, the General Nursing Council is able to assess the number of students who fail to become State Registered and also to keep a check on those who break their training and recommence.

Whitley Councils

The Whitley Council for Nurses and Midwives was inaugurated after the new National Health Service came into being, replacing the Rushcliffe Committee's work of collective bargaining in conditions of service and salary scales.

To the new student it is essential to realise that membership of one or other of the Professional Nursing Organisations gives one the right to bring matters which give rise to discontent to the notice of the organisation, which will, in due course, bring the matter to the correct Committee of the Whitley Council. All the present improvements in salary scales have been brought about by consultations between the staff side (that is us!) and the management, and the council is so constructed that almost completely balanced staff and management sides ensures a fair hearing to all matters brought before the Council.

Professional Nursing Organisations

It is almost essential today that every nurse join one of the Professional Nursing Organisations, since all improvements in conditions of service and pay are brought about through these organisations. They also serve as a link between nurses of other nations, offer facilities for further post-registration education by means of scholarships, or run courses of lectures and even arrange facilities for studying nursing conditions abroad. Most of the organisations have a central club where members may meet both socially and professionally and many happy hours may be spent there.

1. THE ROYAL BRITISH NURSES' ASSOCIATION is at 194 Queen's Gate, London, and was founded in 1887. It has its own journal; it provides a home for the aged nurse. It has its own General Council and, as medical men are permitted to join this Association, has both nurses and medical men on the Committee.

2. THE ROYAL COLLEGE OF NURSING.—Founded in 1916, granted a Royal Charter in 1928 and has a Student Nurses' Association. The Royal College of Nursing is a very active association and although membership fees have gone up to £8 per annum, it ensures the member against any claim for damages which may be brought against him or her in his or her professional capacity. Many courses are run by the College for members and non-members and many students from overseas come to England to take the College courses. The Headquarters are in Henrietta Place, Cavendish Square, London, but branches will be found in almost every town in the British Isles, though the Education Centres are in London, Birmingham and Edinburgh.

In 1962 the Royal College of Nursing and the National Council of Nurses amalgamated forming the Royal College of Nursing and National Council of Nurses of Great Britain and Northern Ireland (now known as Rcn), to represent the voice of the professional nurse, man or woman, both nationally and internationally.

A very active part is taken by the Rcn in the negotiations on the Whitley Council, and is fully representative of all trained nurses—both male and female. The Rcn now publishes its own paper known as the *Nursing Standard*.

THE STUDENT NURSES' ASSOCIATION consists only of Student

Nurses and elects its own committee, honorary officers, president and vice-president and plans its own professional, social, educational and inter-unit activities, and is now part of Rcn.

There are many units of the Association in recognised Training Schools for Nurses in Great Britain and Ireland. They take part in negotiating better conditions and salaries and take an active part in the organisation. The subscription for membership is £1 which covers the three years of training.

3. THE BRITISH COLLEGE OF NURSES.—Founded by Mrs Bedford Fenwick in 1926, in Queen's Gate (number 19). Only general trained Nurses may join. Like the College of Nursing, it aims at furthering the education of the Nurse. Its journal is the *British Journal of Nursing*.

4. STATE ENROLLED NURSES.—Since October 1st 1970, State Enrolled Nurses have full membership of the Rcn. Equally pupils have membership of the Student Nurses Association.

State Enrolled Nurse Regulations

The State Enrolled Nurses Bill was passed in 1943 and amended in 1961, and the General Nursing Council for England and Wales is responsible for enforcing the regulations.

The training of the Pupil Nurse is of two years' duration and a basic training is laid down. An assessment is held by the General Nursing Council after the completion of at least 18 months training. At the end of two years, having passed the assessment, the nurse may apply to be a State Enrolled Nurse. Only certain Training Schools are recognised for Pupil Nurse Training. This Roll of Nurses is of great value to the men or women whose circumstances or knowledge would make it difficult for them to reach the standard required for State Registration. The course is much simpler, theoretically. The enrolled nurse is playing an increasingly important part in fulfilling the nursing needs of the community. Many opportunities are now available for post-enrolment education to fit the nurse for work in specialised fields of nursing, *e.g.* ophthalmic, orthopaedic, domiciliary. The enrolled nurse also makes an important contribution to geriatric nursing.

ETHICS AND HOSPITAL ETIQUETTE

The science of moral conduct is called ethics. Morals are concerned with character and with the distinction between right and wrong. Etiquette is a code of good manners or behaviour practised for the benefit of others or it may be called courtesy. Hospital etiquette is that behaviour which is traditional to hospital life and may be said to 'oil the wheels'. Newcomers will find that it differs very little from the social good manners they were taught in childhood.

A person with suitable qualities who wishes to nurse will have chosen a profession which is of real value to the community and of great satisfaction to one's self. Although the demands are exacting and the standards high, the prospects are excellent, *e.g.* Public Health Nursing, Occupational Health Nursing, The Armed Services, Travel abroad.

PHYSICALLY a nurse must have good health, he or she should be quick and quiet in their actions. They need a pleasant voice and expression and to be dextrous and gentle.

MENTALLY a nurse must be alert and observant and have a good memory for detail. A sound basic education is also essential.

MORALLY a nurse must be reliable and worthy of respect.

These attributes must be applied to a nurse's many duties and are best thought of under definite headings:—

1. TO THE PATIENT.—The primary rule of nursing should be 'Patients first'. Therefore all activities in the ward should be directed to this purpose. A nurse who is tired and harassed may find it helpful to imagine it is one of his or her parents or friends in the patient's place.

Patients should be kept occupied and happy in a quiet manner, the nurse being cheerful and friendly without becoming familiar. Kindly discipline should be maintained and this requires great tact.

It is important for their self respect that patients are addressed by their correct names and adults should be given their appropriate titles, Mr, Mrs or Miss.

2. TO THE PATIENTS' VISITORS.—These people must receive sympathetic courtesy at all times as they are often very distressed and nervous about the condition of their relatives and friends. Questions asked by them should be referred to sister in charge of the ward, as a junior nurse is not really in a position to give appropriate answers.

Gifts from patients and visitors. It is desirable that patients should realise that individual gifts to members of the staff are quite unnecessary, and some patients seeing gifts being given, may be embarrassed, realising that they are not in a position to do the same. Moreover it can lead to misunderstanding, as one patient may feel that his neighbour can 'buy' better attention by his gifts. If, however, a strong desire to give a present is expressed, then it should be done through the hospital authorities and not to any nurse personally.

3. TO SENIOR OFFICERS.—(a) On duty, the nurse's bearing towards medical officers must be strictly professional, addressing them courteously. The nurse must be loyally obedient to the medical staff, remembering that faith in the treatment goes a long way towards the patient's recovery. The medical officers depend greatly on the nurse's powers of observation and precise clear reports.

(b) The nurse must be loyal, polite and obedient to Matron and other senior members of the nursing staff. It will be found easier to obey orders of trained staff implicitly if the student or pupil realises that the nurse in charge of the ward carries responsibility for the actions of all those working under him or her. At the same time, seniors have an obligation to be thoughtful for and courteous to their juniors.

All nursing staff from Matron down to the most junior nurse should be addressed by their proper titles, *e.g.* Matron, Sister, Nurse.

Punctuality is important and the nurse should make a habit of scrutinising various notice boards and making him or herself familiar with any requests made.

4. TO HIS OR HER COLLEAGUES.—A good nurse should be a good work mate, realising that community life has many pleasures but also carries many obligations. He or she should take his or her full share of duty and responsibility and try to be especially helpful and loyal to all his or her colleagues, be they inexperienced senior officers or frightened beginners. He or she will be well behaved, quiet and considerate in the nurses' home and contribute whenever he or she can to the social activities provided. He or she will treat the domestic staff in home and wards with courtesy and thoughtfulness, remembering how dependent he or she will often be on their work and help.

5. TO THE PROFESSION.—On entering the training school a nurse assumes responsibility for the good name not only of the hospital, but for the profession as a whole. Information which he or she acquires professionally, whether it is related to a patient's private affairs or illness, must be kept confidential. Information to the press is usually handled by one of the lay secretaries, and permission must always be obtained from the patient first. The wearing of outdoor uniform should be with care and completeness, that is, coat and hat or cap, gloves and immaculate footwear. The wearer should try to behave in a becoming manner, being quiet and dignified at all times. Conversation in public places such as

restaurants, trains, omnibuses and cinemas should be guarded. It is most improper to discuss diseases, patients and hospital procedures generally. These subjects should also not be discussed in nurses' dining-rooms. Discussion is desirable, but it should be carried on in the seclusion of the nurses' own quarters.

It is also wiser for nurses to choose friends from contemporaries and not amongst those personnel who are very much senior or junior, so avoiding complications when working in the same ward or department.

6. TO THE COMMUNITY.—As a nurse is usually employed under the National Health Service he or she is a public servant. This is a great responsibility, and he or she should learn to serve the community to the best of his or her ability. One of his or her chief responsibilities is to practise economy, see Chapter 2—Hospital Economy.

7. TO HIM OR HERSELF.—Nurses should keep themselves fit mentally and physically as far as possible. This they owe, not only to themselves, but to their patients, employers and colleagues.

Notes on Personal Health are included in their training, and if these are carried out, they will be able to resist infection.

Nurses' uniform is made of washable materials and should always be neat and clean. It is generally considered becoming when properly worn, with neat hairstyles and brightly polished shoes. No jewellery should be worn on duty as it is out of place with uniform and may harbour bacteria and damage patients' skin when treatments are carried out.

Finally, nurses owe it to themselves and the community to become as well qualified and informed as possible. They should listen to lectures carefully and be ready to participate in discussions and debates, thus acquiring a thorough understanding of the subject. They should use reference books so that their work is accurate and free from spelling mistakes, and they should arrange their work neatly and methodically.

Nurses should do as much professional reading as possible and 'read up' special cases. Some time should be set aside for quiet thought about lectures and experience gained.

Nurses must learn to be observant and to give clear reports as well as trying at all times to improve their dexterity and skill, and understand that as long as they are in active employment their training and learning never ceases.

LEGAL ASPECTS FOR NURSES

The hospital is liable to pay damages to anyone who is injured, through carelessness or incompetence of any member of the staff. The hospital liability does not absolve the member from blame and he or she also is liable to be sued.

If, however, a patient suffers injury or accident, which is not the result of carelessness, then there is no liability on the part of the hospital or nurse.

If a patient falls out of bed or sustains any other injury (which may or may not be the result of carelessness) however minor, he or she must be seen by a medical officer, and an accident form filled in accurately, because if the patient dies within a year, an inquest will have to be held.

PATIENT'S WILLS

Patients often wish to make a will during their stay in hospital, and a solicitor may be needed. It is a rule of most hospitals that *no member* of the nursing staff should witness a will, but are in duty bound to fetch someone who can, *e.g.* a member of the hospital secretarial staff.

POINTS TO REMEMBER IN HOSPITAL

1. Attend to visitors promptly and pleasantly.
2. Patients' friends are admitted at stated visiting times, or by arrangement with the Sister or nurse in charge.
3. Sister or nurse in charge should be informed immediately any medical or nursing staff, hospital staff, committee members, chaplains or other people, enter the ward.
4. When going through swing doors, make sure no one is following immediately behind.
5. Always add the appropriate title if possible when replying to instructions.
6. Messages accepted by a junior nurse should be conveyed accurately.
7. Nurses should report on and off duty and before and after meals to Sister or nurse in charge. There may be messages or instructions to be given.
8. Seats should be provided for those wishing to speak to patients.
9. When tending a patient in company with a colleague, it is courteous and kind to include the patient in any conversations.
10. Wards, sluices, corridors and staircases should be kept as quiet as possible by the wearing of soft rubber heels, careful handling

of stainless steel, crockery, cutlery, doors, etc., and by essential talking being carried on in as quiet a voice as possible.
11. Uniform should be complete, neat and clean. When outdoor uniform is not provided, mufti coats and hats should not be worn over uniform dresses. Uniform is the property of the hospital and the responsibility of the individual to whom it is issued. It should not be loaned or borrowed.
12. Suede shoes are unsuitable for nursing duties.
13. Nurses should write to Matron, if it is impossible to return from holiday or sick leave at the correct time.
14. Nurses should report to Home Sister on return from holidays or sick leave, and to Matron's Office next day at office time.
15. See that the Sisters know the times and dates of examinations, if they occur while on duty.
16. Report to Home Sister in the event of indisposition or illness *however slight*. *Any* member of the nursing staff falling sick at home, whether resident or non-resident, must *immediately* send a message to the hospital, so that arrangements can be made to provide a relief. A written message should be marked 'URGENT' and addressed to Matron. In this case, whoever is on duty in the Nursing Administration Office can open the message and deal with the matter. A telephone message should be sent to Matron, or whoever is on duty. There is always someone on duty for her, day and night, weekends or holidays.
17. Go to wards and departments only when sent or when given special permission, apart from actual duties.
18. Cloaks are intended for outdoor use, but may be used indoors if building is particularly cold.
19. Radio sets in the Nurses' Home should be turned low, so that other residents will not be unkindly disturbed. Clicking heels, loud talking and laughter should be controlled in the corridors for the same reason. Baths should not be turned on after 10.30 p.m. when the Home should be quite quiet for the benefit of those who wish to sleep.

THE PSYCHOLOGICAL ASPECT OF NURSING

A hospital is a place in which patients are treated and nursed, and persons who wish to become good nurses will never for one moment forget that the first and main function of the hospital is the care and cure of the patients. They will soon learn that illness and separation from normal surroundings give rise to abnormality, and they will find many patients trying, and many nursing details unpleasant. Enthusiastic, sympathetic nurses will, however, find ways and means of understanding and overcoming these difficulties.

When relatives bring a patient into hospital, they come with very mixed feelings; fear of the outcome of the treatment, fear of the strange, unfamiliar surroundings and sorrow at the enforced separation. Cheerful, friendly, helpful nurses will instil hope and courage, where possibly efficient but unfriendly and bustling persons will still further depress their low spirits.

Where the patient is the bread-winner for the family, or the mother of young children, the worries of both patient and relatives are intensified. The most pitiable subject, however, is probably a small child, unable to understand the need for treatment. To minimise the trauma involved, most hospitals have the facilities for a mother to stay with her child while in hospital, helping with the care necessary, and maintaining a continuity and feeling of security experienced at home.

The adult patient, though able to understand the need for the treatment, is less adaptable to his surroundings. The unfamiliar bed, the unfamiliar meals and routine are very trying. Nurses with any imagination and sympathy will do their utmost to secure the patient's privacy on all occasions, by the use of curtains or screens, and take care not to expose the patient more than is absolutely essential.

Then again the ill patient will be helpless, and therefore entirely dependent on an ever-changing series of strange young people for every attention, a situation that has not before been endured since babyhood. The efficient, impersonal, yet kindly care of the nurses can do much to make the unpleasant situation tolerable.

Nurses who have sufficient imagination and sympathy to picture themselves in the position of the patient and of his relatives are the so-called 'born nurses' or as they are called today 'psychologically minded'. It means nurses who are interested in, and anxious to understand, the workings of the human mind, and particularly those of their patients, their relatives, their colleagues and themselves. They will soon learn how physical suffering reacts on the mind, disturbing the will and emotions in such a way that the patient does not behave as he would under normal conditions.

Nurses with the gift of making their patients feel at ease and free from fear, inspire confidence and provide an atmosphere of peace and security so necessary for relaxation of mind and body, an important factor in the treatment of disease.

Relationship between nurse and patient

The psychological factor may not be consciously appreciated by the nurses, but it is present in the performance of many of their routine duties, *e.g.*

1. Patience in persuading a patient to take food or medicine.
2. Confidence when persuading a patient to accept treatment.
3. Tact and kindness in performing intimate duties.

In these and many other ways nurses can inspire their patients with confidence, trust and hope.

Responsibilities of a nurse to her patients

The sort of discipline expected in hospitals results in good team work and in *safeguarding human life*.

Rules controlling the safe custody and administration of dangerous drugs and poisons must be rigidly adhered to, or mistakes with fatal consequences may occur.

Rules governing aseptic technique must be carried out with meticulous care in order to prevent infection. A patient's life may easily rest on the conscientious work of a nurse in the operating theatre.

Nurses are in charge of patients' lives, a very great and arduous responsibility, yet a very great privilege, since the patients' relatives leave them in our care with hope, and our reward lies in their recovery, or at least in the alleviation of their sufferings, and the immense satisfaction of knowing that our work, whatever its nature, helped. The joy and gratitude of those who recover, and the thanks of the relatives of those whom we can only assist, make every effort worthwhile.

Influence on environment in illness

While in hospital patients miss their usual surroundings very much, the people with whom they live and work, and their treasured possessions and animals. A nurse should endeavour to compensate the patient for this loss by making his life and surroundings in hospital as happy and cheerful as possible under the circumstances, *e.g.* Ward Sisters will often try to put patients in beds next to patients who will be congenial companions.

A cheerful and happy staff, bright flowers, pretty bed covers, light coloured walls, etc., all help.

Relationship between nurse and patient's relatives and friends

Relatives and friends are often over-anxious and fearful of leaving the patient. They are generally too worried to listen accurately to instructions. Whenever possible *written* instructions relating to telephone calls or enquiries should be given, when kindly neighbours will often deal with the matter. Considerable patience, tact, sympathy and understanding are required in dealing with relatives and friends. Nurses should avoid any tendency to become possessive and must remember that the patient belongs to his relatives and friends. They have *every right* to enquire and visit him whenever possible. If, owing to the exigencies of the ward work, it is impossible for them to see him, the fact must be carefully and *sympathetically* explained and the reasons given. Relatives must be made to feel that their enquiries are welcome and will be conveyed to the patient. Nurses should do all in their power to reassure them and give good news of progress made. If, however, there is little hope of recovery, the Doctor or Ward Sister will explain the expected outcome as kindly as possible, making it clear, so that they can prepare themselves accordingly, should the patient die.

THE NURSE IN RELATION TO THE TEACHING OF HEALTH

Nurses have many opportunities of teaching the principles of health. They can set a good example by the way they live themselves. They should display physical and mental poise, refraining from vulgarity and behaving with dignity. Their quiet, confident manners, personal fastidiousness and general tidiness, will all contribute to inspiring confidence. They should always show an interest in questions or remarks addressed to them. Nurses should always be courteous and considerate to others. These qualities in a nurse's character determine the amount of influence they will be able to exercise in a community of actual or potential patients, and the degree of respect and confidence they can command.

Continuance of this influence and respect will depend on:

1. Care of other people's possessions.
2. Working in a thorough, tidy, methodical way.
3. Punctuality.
4. Being economical.
5. Leaving no unnecessary clearing-up for others.
6. Courtesy to colleagues and *all grades* of workers.

Nurses on duty in a hospital ward or department are always being observed by the patient. If they are vulgar, noisy, untidy, careless or unpunctual, they will not only be a public disgrace, but no patient will respect them. It would not be wise to retain such nurses on the hospital staff. On the other hand, keen nurses, neat and fresh in appearance, thorough and tidy in their work, punctual, careful of other people's possessions, dignified, courteous and pleasant, will not only set a good example, but will inspire respect and confidence, and be an asset to any community.

Relatives, friends and neighbours and casual acquaintances will all approach nurses for advice on health, partly because of their practical experience, and partly because they are more easily approached than a doctor.

After training as a nurse, Public Health work, lecturing to Red Cross and St John's organisations, and to Youth Clubs, affords great scope for contacting more people and educating them in the principles of health.

Whenever possible, nurses should point out how important it is for *each individual* to contribute materially to the sound health of the community in which the person lives.

Factors which contribute to breakdown in health

1. Fatigue.
2. Constant background of noise.
3. Insufficient or unsuitable food.
4. Bad cooking.
5. Hurried meals.
6. Poor ventilation.
7. Inadequate or unsuitable clothing.
8. Badly fitting shoes.
9. Over-crowding.
10. Faulty housing.
11. Over-strain or unsuitable occupation.
12. Bad habits; *e.g.* excessive smoking.

With the increase of medical knowledge and separation of diseases into special groups, practically every organ in man's body is dealt with by a specialist. The nurse, however, deals with all patients, whatever their disease, as a whole individual having a mind as well as a body.

Because the range of nursing is so great, considerable knowledge, acquired through training, in addition to their natural qualities, is needed in order that they may control their own lives wisely and exert good influence on others.

As nurses serve the people from babyhood to the grave they learn the tragedies that can occur in families when responsibilities of family life are neglected.

In the struggle for health nurses can prepare for the fight against disease by teaching preventive measures by example and precept. They can also teach first aid and hygiene. Some nurses will be able to help people to rehabilitate themselves after severe illness or accident; others will be caring for those who are mentally or emotionally upset.

Nurses who are engaged in caring for those who are ill or infirm can by their thoughtfulness and understanding, alter the feeling of embarrassment and anxiety which is often felt by a patient in hospital, to confidence and tranquillity. They can turn chaos and dread of illness in a family into order and courage so that the trouble can be met with calm and strength.

There is great scope for nurses as missionaries and teachers of health in undeveloped communities, where there is a need for nursing and medical services. In all parts of the world, and among all colours, creeds and types who require their services, nurses carry on their work.

When they take into account a patient's occupation and interests, both economic and family, as well as carrying out bedside nursing, they are practising nursing in the true sense of the word, and can estimate the value of human life. This knowledge is transmitted back to the patient by teaching him how to preserve health.

If nurses understand community life and its problems, they are in a position to take matters of health to the proper authorities, so linking it up with environment and preventive action.

Through their professional organisations they are linked to the International Council of Nurses; by this means they are able to meet nurses of other countries.

Nurses may perform many social and civic duties and by their interests can convert apathy into activity. They may form groups and clubs for the young, speak to housewives, encourage old and lonely people to have constructive ideas and form clubs where their interests may be developed. They can explain medical and nursing information heard on the radio, at talks and lectures, or read in newspapers and magazines.

They can encourage many young people to take up nursing by giving an outline of their own training days and the happiness they experienced.

Chapter Two

THE WARD AND ANNEXES

General Management—Cleaning and care of equipment—Economy

GENERAL MANAGEMENT

VENTILATION.—The ward should be airy, windows open as necessary, draughts avoided.

LIGHTING.—The windows are usually arranged in relation to beds to ensure maximum amount of light. Artificial lighting is carried out by means of large central lights, with individual lights over beds. Anglepoise or bell-lamps are used for treatments if necessary. Arrangements are made for night lighting either by special bulb (red or blue) in central lights or by shading lights over beds, and nowadays lights can be dimmed at the switch, especially in side wards. This enables the constant observation of the critically ill patients.

HEATING.—This is usually carried out by central heating apparatus; radiators are controllable. Occasionally electric, gas or coal fires are available for convalescent patients to sit by. They should be well guarded.

Temperature of ward should be 65° F. Sister will notify engineer if unsatisfactory.

NOISE IN HOSPITAL.—Can retard the patients' recovery by causing irritation and sleeplessness. Little can be done about the increasing noise from road, rail or air traffic, building operations and roadworks, or, at night, about patients who moan and snore in their sleep. Other sources of noise can, however, be reduced. Nursing staff should move in a composed way and not rush heavily in clattering shoes on hard floors. Metal bedpans on metal trolleys or racks are ear piercing, polypropylene or fibre glass might be substituted, and metal bowls or enamel mugs could also be eliminated. Doors and trolley wheels can be oiled. Cupboard and locker doors should not be fitted with spring catches. Hissing sterilisers and dripping taps can be dealt with. At night, whispering and creeping round a ward should be avoided. Nursing staff should set a good example to domestic helpers by handling plates and cutlery as quietly as possible. Efforts are being made to produce vacuum cleaners and electric scrubbers which make less noise. In new hospitals it is to be hoped that sluices, kitchens, stores and lifts will be shut off from the patients and that noisy metal equipment will be replaced with quieter material.

ROUTINE.—Ward management includes careful planning of the routine work. Many patients find that they are extremely busy with little time for rest. Baths, toiletting, temperatures, dressings, medicines, meals, doctors rounds, getting up, visits by the Medical Social Worker, laboratory staff, occupational therapist, and friends completely fill the day. Much research has been done on this subject recently, and the Department of Health issued a helpful report called the 'Pattern of the In-patient's Day'. The habits of people in different areas vary tremendously, however, so it is necessary for each hospital nursing administrative staff to work out its own satisfactory routine, taking local conditions into account. They are, however, all agreed that patients should not be wakened too early in the morning. Seven a.m. has been suggested as a suitable time.

CLEANING

A nurse must know the proper methods of cleaning so that she may be competent to keep the patient's sickroom in a condition of cleanliness, essential to his welfare and comfort, *should no domestic help be available*. Most hospitals now have domestic supervisors to relieve the nursing staff of the responsibility of all non-nursing duties.

Rules:
1. Collect all articles required before commencing work.
2. Brooms, dusters, polishers and water must be clean.
3. Sweep first, except for high dusting, with a proper brush, of walls, ledges and blinds.
4. Dusting should be done with a damp duster—polished surfaces dried afterwards with a soft dry duster. Dust from top to bottom of article using firm even strokes.
5. All rubbish must be removed from tables and lockers (with patient's permission) when dusting. Scrub and tidy insides of lockers weekly for long-term patients.
6. Furniture (including locker tops and bed-tables) should be polished once a week using furniture cream sparingly.
7. Paintwork should be washed with soapy water, cleaning powder used only to remove marks.
8. Use all cleaning materials with care and economy.

All cleaning should be carried out quietly and with as little disturbance of patients as possible, using method and thoroughness, returning furniture to its rightful place.

It is desirable that vacuum cleaners should be used for all cleaning.

WALLS.—Usually washable—either paint or tiles. Dust with wall brush. Periodically washed by male cleaners.
Wash theatre walls daily.

FLOORS.—*Stone, cement, tiled or mosaic.* Scrub with soapy water, rinse and dry well. *Composition, rubber or linoleum.* Wash with soapy water; rinse and dry well (*N.B.* Special mops and electric scrubbers now available.) *Wood Blocks.* Polish with electric polishers; occasionally washed. Water spilt must be wiped up immediately; it is dangerous because it makes the floor slippery and spoils polished surface. Ideally, vacuum cleaners are used; if not available, mops impregnated with a special oil are often used.

It is strongly advised that a 'shoe-bath', *i.e.* a sheet of foam rubber soaked with suitable germicidal detergent such as Hibitane, should be placed at entrances to departments, *e.g.* operating theatres.

ELECTRIC LIGHTS.—Dust daily if within reach. Centre lights washed periodically.

Caution.—Turn off electricity when dusting with damp duster or changing bulbs. Shades should be plain to facilitate cleaning and prevent collection of dust.

METAL.—*Brass and copper.* Clean with metal polish, unless lacquered. *Chromium plating and stainless steel.* Wash with soapy water; rinse and dry with clean duster.

WOODWORK.—*Unpolished.* Scrub along grain with soap and water; rinse and dry as well as possible. *Polished.* Furniture cream should be applied once a week; a wash leather may be used first if necessary.

GLASS.—Wash with leather or soap and water; rinse and polish with dry duster or newspaper.

TROLLEY AND SCREEN WHEELS.—Scrape and oil periodically.

WARD KITCHEN.—Use gas and electricity with care. Turn off when not required.

General cleaning of kitchen, including stoves and hot plates, is carried out by domestic assistant, but food spilt must be wiped up immediately, and soiled utensils neatly stacked to minimise work.

Saucepans.—Put to soak in cold water after use. Special saucepans reserved for milk.

Crockery.—All crockery and utensils must be washed thoroughly. Nurses responsibility to see that it is all spotless when given out to patients.

Feeding cups.—Clean spouts with special brush.

Cruets.—Clean and keep filled.

Infectious crockery.—Disposable utensils are used *i.e.* plates.

Refrigerators.—Wash out daily, replace articles on correct shelves.

Cupboard and larder shelves.—Scrub and replace articles correctly. Cover all food. Return unwanted food to central kitchen. Put waste food in pig bucket (no egg-shells, tins, tea leaves, paper, etc.). When stacking plates, scrape left-overs into bowl on trolley; stand cutlery in jug of water.

General repairs, e.g. dripping taps. Report to Sister; dealt with by appropriate department.

WARD BATHROOM, STERILISING ROOM, LAVATORY AND SLUICE ROOM.—*Baths and sinks.* Clean daily with cleaning powder. Pay special attention to parts under taps, overflow and waste outlet, use old pair of forceps for removing waste that tends to clog latter.

Washing bowls, tooth mugs and vomit bowls.—Clean with powder after each use. Boil tooth mugs if possible. Tooth mugs are often disposable.

Sterilisers.—Empty, clean and rinse before use each morning. Clean dresssing bowls and dishes with powder before sterilising.

Dirty dressing bins.—Desirable that these be dealt with in a central station, if staff, space and equipment available. Otherwise, after being emptied by porters, should be mopped out with disinfectant, *e.g.* Izal 1 : 40, rinsed and turned upside down to drain; may then be lined with a waxed paper bag before use. More frequently nowadays, disposable waterproof bags are used.

Bedpan washers, sluices and lavatory pans. Sprinkle with Harpic or suitable disinfectant, leave at least half an hour, then scrub with special brush and flush. Brush should be kept in enamel holder containing Jeyes fluid 1 : 40. Wash and dry seats of lavatory pans on both sides.

Bedpans, urinals and chambers. Flush with cold water after use; then mop with hot water and rinse. In some hospitals, bedpan sterilisers are provided and bedpans are boiled for five minutes after each round.

Sputum mugs. Empty and flush with cold water (contents measured first, if necessary). Wash in hot soapy water using mop and boil for five minutes in special steriliser or pan.

Special apparatus used for dealing with mugs in sanatoria. Mugs may have waxed linings or destructible cartons may be used.

Removal of stains from linen

1. *Blood. Soak in cold water.* If stain dried into material, hydrogen peroxide or ammonia may be used; rinse afterwards.
2. *Ink.* Soak article at once in cold water or milk. Prolonged soaking may be necessary, *e.g.* twenty-four hours.
3. *Tea, coffee, cocoa.* Wash in cold water; then pour boiling water on stain. Bleaching agent may be used, rinse well.

4. *Fruit stains.* Rub with salt, then treat as above.
5. *Rust marks.* Difficult to remove, but may be possible with salt and lemon juice and exposure to sunlight.

Removal of vomit or excreta from floor

Cover with sand or sawdust. Remove with dustpan and brush which can be washed afterwards. Mop floor.
or
Clean up with newspaper which can be burnt. Mop floor.

HOSPITAL ECONOMY

Cotton materials of all kinds, including lint, gauze, bandages and cotton wool are expensive and it is important that they are used only where no other substitute will suffice, and even then as sparingly as possible.

1. Dressings should be cut exactly to required size, nowadays are often supplied commercially prepared.
2. Lint or other dressing material must never be used for cleaning or as dusters.
3. Patients should be encouraged to provide own toilet flannels, so that lint is not used for this purpose. Emergency admissions usually provided with disposable flannels which can be used a number of times.
4. Waxed bags used for soiled dressings, should not be used for parcels.
5. Bandages should always be carefully removed, washed and ironed or rolled, to be used several times.
6. Care should be exercised to prevent ink, iodine or other stains dropping on bed linen, patients' clothing, nurses' uniforms or floors. If such should happen, immediate steps should be taken to remove stain.
7. Gauze plugging is specially prepared and is expensive; it should not be used for finger bandages or to tie up parcels.
8. Splints are provided already padded, with waterproof covering.
9. Garments (including uniform) or linen in need of repair, tapes or buttons should be put aside for repairs; they should not be kept in use until the damage is irreparable.
10. If garments must be cut to cope with a patient's particular disability, *e.g.* arm splint, they must be carefully cut along the seams. Special garments are sometimes available or other arrangements can be made.
11. Soiled linen must be transported in proper containers, *i.e*

disposable plastic bags, canvas bags or wicker baskets; it should never be tied up in a sheet or counterpane.
12. Wet linen must be dried immediately; if put aside wet, mildew will appear on articles in contact with it.
13. Napkins, if properly used to protect patients' garments and bed linen during meal times, will prevent unnecessarily frequent laundering.
14. Special articles of linen must be used only for purpose for which they are intended in the interests both of economy and cleanliness.
15. Bed linen caught on mattress wire must be gently freed; care should be taken not to tear; if necessary, bedstead should be put aside for attention.
16. Bedclothes should not touch floor when beds are stripped.
17. If blankets are needed next to patient, they should be of flannelette washable variety.
18. Pillows must be adequately protected from discharges, etc., by means of a plastic pillow case.
19. All bedding must be carefully protected when sent for disinfection.
20. Leaking taps, gas rings, loose screws, windows, etc., ill-fitting doors and all minor repairs should be reported to Sister at once and by her to the appropriate department.
21. Turn off all gas, electricity and steam whenever possible.
22. Small mops or cloths and detergent powders or liquids should be provided in bathrooms ready for use.
23. Rubber articles must be carefully dried, powdered and, where possible, inflated with air before being put away, or they will perish. Grease, pins and heat must be kept away from rubber articles.
24. Syringes, which are not disposable, should be rinsed immediately after use, so that they will not stick.
25. If a pint of lotion is sufficient, do not prepare three pints, and always prepare accurately as ordered.
26. Medicine, tablets, etc., of patients who have gone home, must be returned at once to the dispensary, not thrown out or used for others.
27. As far as possible order proper quantity of bread and butter, cocoa, etc.; excess amounts generally have to be put in the pig bucket.
28. Milk must be kept in a cool place and boiled if there is any possibility of it turning sour.
29. Breakable objects such as thermometers and glasses must be carefully placed on lockers or tables so that they cannot be knocked off.

30. Lockers must be placed so that patients can use them easily or articles will be dropped, or the patient may overbalance in reaching for something and fall out of bed.
31. See that waste-pipe is kept free. Plumbers spend much time on waste pipes which have become blocked by hair grips, wool, tea leaves, matches, orange peel, razor blades and other oddments.

Equipment

In equipping a ward, allowance should be made for articles broken or awaiting replacement, or for linen and clothes at the laundry and mending room.

EQUIPMENT FOR 100 PATIENTS' BEDS:

Bedding		*Bedclothes*	
Bedsteads	105	Pillow cases	600
Wire mattress covers	105	Counterpanes	160
Mattresses	110	Blankets	500
Mattress covers	110	Sheets	600
Pillows	350	Draw sheets	600
Pillow covers	350		

House Linen

Bath towels	250	Hand towels	400

Chapter Three

BEDMAKING

Care of beds and bedding, linen—Routine and special bedmaking —Positions used—Bed accessories—Filling hot water bottles

BEDS

Bedstead

Modern hospital bedstead. Enamelled iron or aluminium, 6 ft. 3 ins. by 3 ft. by 2 ft. 3 ins. high. Lends uniformity. Facilitates treatment; easily made and kept clean; patient away from ground draughts. Castors or wheels give mobility; a brake gives security. There are many adjustable beds now in use *e.g.* Hilo beds.

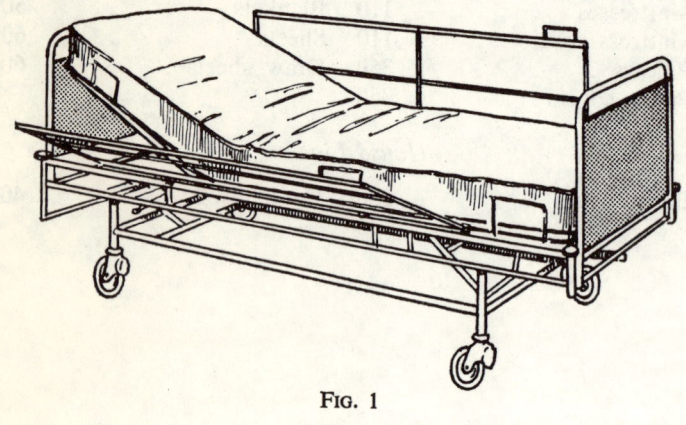

FIG. 1
Hilo bed.

Mattress frame

Wire-sprung.
To clean.—Dust with damp cloth.
To disinfect.—Mop thoroughly with Bradosol 1:2000 or other disinfectant.

Mattress

1. Horsehair, protected by plastic cover. Turn when bed is made, if possible, to ensure even wear.

2. Interior sprung, protected by plastic cover. Turn once a week.
3. Sorbo, covered with polythene covers. Do not turn unless double thickness.

Pillows

Flock or horsehair for support | Protect with plastic cover
   Feather for comfort | if necessary.
   Dunlopillo and latex foam pillows.

Blankets

1. White wool or cellular cotton used for general bedmaking.
2. Coloured, used for top blanket. Also for getting patient up and taking to various departments.
3. Grey blankets, used for admission of dirty patient, *e.g.* road accident.
4. Flannelette, used for admission and bath.
5. Flannelette, or old thin blankets used for inside blankets.

All bedding is kept clean by use of vacuum cleaners. Signs of wear and tear should be reported and attended to immediately.

To disinfect.—Submit to steam under pressure in an autoclave (10 lbs. for 20 mins.), or fumigate.

LINEN

Varieties of linen

COUNTERPANES.—Light in colour and weight, of uniform pattern.
SHEETS.—Cotton or linen or mixture of both. Linen wears well, looks nice, but is expensive and cold.
DRAW SHEETS.—Twilled cotton, warmer and more absorbent. Twice width of bed in length. From patient's mid-back to knees in width. Used for protection of large sheets. Draw sheets are not used nowadays, unless patient is incontinent, and then they may be protected by incontinence pads. They may also be used where there is a risk of soiling or if the patient is hot and sticky.

To disinfect linen

Linen is put into special waterproof plastic bags and sent to the laundry, where it is put straight into a special machine.

Laundry arrangements recommended by the Department of Health

Three types of linen to be dealt with:

1. Ordinary soiled linen from bed changing.
2. Linen from infectious patients.
3. Linen fouled by incontinent patients.

It is firmly recommended that no soiled linen should be counted in wards or departments and that linen and blankets be put straight into strong canvas bags or nylon bags when removed from the beds. The bags could be marked or coloured to denote category of linen. The bags must be sealed before removal from wards or departments and only opened in sorting room.

It is also recommended that the sluicing of fouled linen by hand should cease. It should be sent in special containers, appropriately marked, to a central sluicing department.

Infected linen should be sent to the laundry in specially marked containers.

Soiled linen should be removed regularly from the wards and departments, but it is advisable that it should not be transported along main corridors and in patients' lifts.

Washing and sterilising blankets

Blankets must be washed and sterilised regularly, *i.e.* after each discharge of short stay patients and each week for long stay patients. They may be safely and adequately washed and sterilised by the use of Lissapol N (a non-ionic detergent) and Cirrasol, or similar preparations.

Care of linen

1. Store in heated cupboards with racked shelves.
2. Arrange in groups of like kind, so that linen is easily collected and used in rotation.
3. Send to laundry before it is too dirty, removing stains first.
4. Use small pieces to protect larger items, *e.g.* draw sheets, napkins.
5. Use items only for the purpose for which they are intended.
6. Torn linen must never be used on beds.

Most hospitals have a system of central linen supply with a 'topping up' system. All checking and mending is done in the linen room and is not the responsibility of the nurses.

BEDMAKING

General rules

1. Have everything at hand before commencing.
2. Strip bed neatly, clothes not touching the floor, handle bedclothes carefully, avoid flapping to minimise risk of cross infection by spreading dust. Have chair or 'bed stripper' near for pillows and accessories.
3. Keep patient in position required for his treatment throughout.
4. Keep patient well covered with blanket.
5. Support patient when necessary. One nurse may do this as other makes one side of bed.
6. Strip to bottom of bed, always removing plastic and cotton draw sheets.
7. Pull mattress well up to bed head.
8. Shake pillows at each making—not over patient's feet. Tuck in ends of cases firmly and replace with open end away from door. Arrange to support patient in comfort.
9. Allow room for patient's feet, when replacing top bed clothes.
10. Call for help when necessary to move heavy or very ill patient.

AN EMPTY BED

Requirements.—Interior sprung mattress with plastic cover.
Or—

Sorbo mattress with plastic case.	Plastic draw sheet.
Hard pillow and pillow case.	2 or 3 blankets.
Soft pillow and pillow case.	Counterpane.
2 sheets.	Cotton draw sheet.

Method:

1. Protect mattress as above.
2. Open bottom sheet, right side uppermost and place evenly on bed.
3. Fix top with mitred corners, fix bottom, pulling tight, with mitred corners, tuck in sides, to make firm foundation.
4. Place plastic draw sheet appropriately to come under patient's buttocks.
5. Place and tuck in cotton draw sheet to cover the above completely, excess on the locker side.
6. Place pillow at head of bed, with the pillow case completely covering the ticking and the open end away from the door.
7. Open top sheet, right side downwards, with top 18 ins. fold

brought halfway up pillow, remainder at bottom tucked in with box corners, together with top blankets.
8. Place first blanket with 6 ins. turn over to come halfway up the pillow after mitring corners, to allow free movement and good chest and shoulder protection. Place remaining blankets, tuck in sides and bottom together with top sheet, using box corners and loosening over feet.
9. Open counterpane and place centrally, turn under top, allowing sufficient to tuck in with mitred corners at bottom.
10. Turn back 18 ins. of top sheet and see that it hangs neatly.
11. Place other pillow over this, with the same care as the first one.
12. Replace chair and locker and align the bed, with castors turned into the head.

AN OCCUPIED BED

TO STRIP THE BED:
1. Place stripper or chair at foot of the bed. Chair at side.
2. Loosen sides and foot of clothes, beginning at top of bed.
3. Turn back top sheet.
4. Remove counterpane by folding into three and placing it on the stripper.
5. Remove blankets in the same way, except for the last one.
6. Remove top sheet beneath blanket, from top to bottom, holding blanket over patient's shoulders with hand nearest head of bed, so that patient is not exposed or subjected to a draught.
Fold sheet in three and place on stripper.

TO MAKE THE BED:

With the patient lying full length:
1. Remove as many pillows as possible, leaving at least one soft pillow under the head. Put pillows on chair.
2. Move the pillow over to the side of the bed towards which you intend to turn the patient.
3. Roll patient to the side under covering blanket, and support.
4. Untuck cotton and plastic draw sheets and roll each close to patient.
5. Untuck bottom sheet and turn back; straighten mattress cover.
6. Replace sheet using mitred corners.
7. Move pillow over to opposite side of bed, roll patient over, freeing the blanket as necessary, keeping the back covered. Support.
8. Remove, shake and fold cotton and plastic draw sheets and place on stripper.
9. Deal with bottom of bed as before.

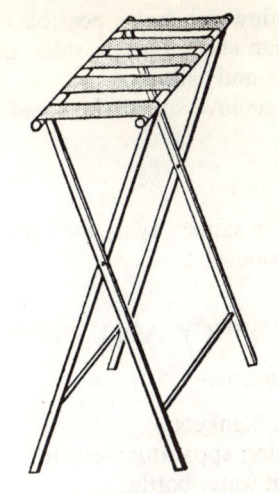

Fig. 2
Bed Stripper.

10. Replace plastic and cotton draw sheets, tucking in excess and rolling free sides towards patient.
11. Roll back patient just enough to free plastic and cotton draw sheets, roll free and tuck in these.
12. Make up bed as before, removing the blanket under the top sheet, loosening blankets over patient's feet.

With the patient moving to foot of bed:

1. Support patient (warmly wrapped in blanket) at foot of bed, making sure rail is protected to prevent patient's legs from being hurt.
2. Remove pillows, cotton and plastic draw sheets.
3. Make top half of foundation of bed, replacing the above.
4. Help patient back to position, keeping him covered.
5. Make up bed as before.

N.B. Bottom sheet and draw sheet may be changed if necessary with patient handled as above, *i.e. side to side,* and *top to bottom.* Clean linen and laundry bag should be available.

To Change Bottom Sheet from Top to Bottom:

1. After stripping, lift patient to foot of bed and support. Protect rail to prevent patient's legs from being hurt.
2. Remove cotton and plastic draw sheets and pillows. Untuck and

roll bottom sheet down as far as possible.
3. Tuck in top of clean sheet, tuck in sides and replace plastic and cotton draw sheets and pillows.
4. Lift patient back, remove soiled sheet and finish bed as above.

Cot making

Cots are made in the same way as the beds, but the counterpane is tucked in on each side.

EMERGENCY ADMISSION BEDS

Additional requirements.—

    2 bath blankets.
    Warming apparatus—electric blanket or hot water bottle.

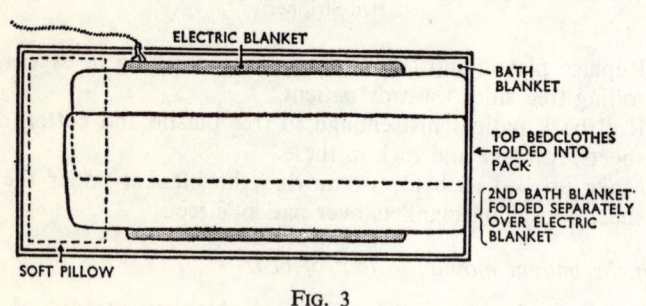

FIG. 3
Prepared bed.

Method:

1. Make foundation of bed as usual, leaving one soft pillow in position.
2. Cover with bath blanket, turning under at sides.
3. Put in electric blanket or hot water bottles, if this is considered necessary *e.g.* elderly patient.
4. Place second bath blanket, folded, over this.
5. Place top bedclothes, folding back at foot. Turn down 18 ins. of top sheet—then fold all into pack of three.

Have available—thermometer tray and chart, consent form, blanket bath trolley, bedpan.

Other articles according to diagnosis and condition of patient.

CARDIAC BEDS

To Make an Acute Cardiac Bed.—Patient nursed flat, at rest, unless dyspnoea is present.

Additional requirements:

>1 soft pillow.
>Inside blanket.
>Cradle and sandbag (covered).

Method:

1. Make foundation of bed as usual.
2. Place one soft pillow under patient's head.
3. Place inside blanket loosely over patient.
4. Support feet with sandbag.
5. Take weight of bedclothes off feet with cradle.
6. Make rest of bed as usual.
7. Carry out 'complete nursing care'.

To Make a Chronic Cardiac Bed.—Patient has chronic heart condition and suffers from dyspnoea or even orthopnoea. He must be nursed in position which supplies maximum comfort and least distress in breathing.

Additional requirements:

>Firm pillows or backrest.
>Soft pillows for comfort.
>Inside blanket.
>Cradle.
>Sandbag and air ring (both covered).
>Chest blanket.
>Heart table.

Method:

1. Arrange pillows to support patient comfortably.
2. Arrange inside blanket loosely, with sandbag at feet. Air ring (covered) if necessary and if desired.
3. Place cradle over inside blanket.
4. Make rest of bed as usual.
5. Place heart table in position, with pillow protected by plastic cover.
6. Have chest blanket at hand to put round patient's shoulders if necessary.

7. Carry out 'complete nursing care'.
8. Have within reach of patient:
>> Sputum mug.
>> Drink (if allowed).
>> Bell (if patient is alone).

N.B.—Cardiac beds which are especially adjustable are often used for these patients nowadays.

POST-OPERATION BED

Additional requirements:
>> Protective sheeting.
>> Towel.
>> Inside blanket.
>> Electric blanket or hot water bottles.

On chair: Pillows or any extra requirements for particular operation, *e.g.* firm pillows, bedrest, plastic covered pillow, sandbags.
Under foot of bed: Elevator.

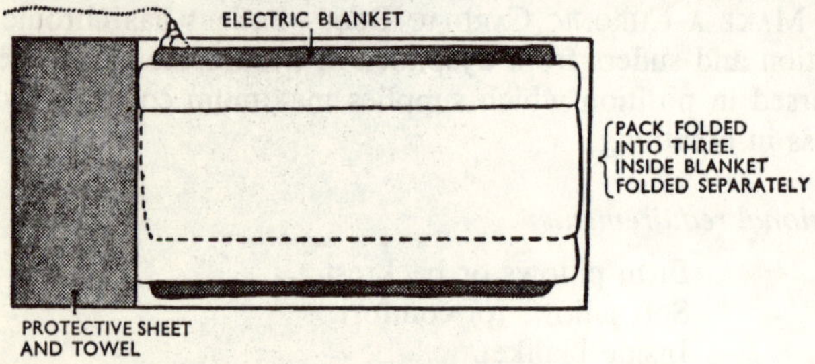

FIG. 4
Prepared bed.

Method:
1. Leave pillows on chair.
2. Make foundation as usual.
3. Place protective sheeting and towel over head of bed and tuck under mattress.
4. Put in electric blanket or hot water bottles. (See note below.)
5. Place inside blanket, folded over this.
6. Put top clothes on as for admission bed, turning up at bottom and then folding into three to form a long pack down centre of bed.
7. Place post-anaesthetic tray and half-hourly pulse chart on locker.
8. Have at hand oxygen cylinder and hypodermic tray.

BEDMAKING

N.B.—Heating apparatus and inside blanket are not always used, nowadays.

Post-anaesthetic tray should be left on locker until patient has recovered from anaesthetic.

On return from theatre the patient must be kept under constant observation until he has regained complete consciousness.

In many hospitals, patients often kept in post-anaesthetic or recovery ward until safe to return to ward.

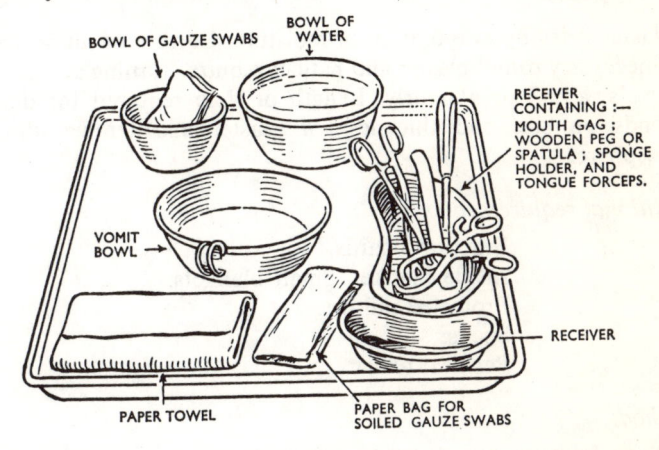

Fig. 5

Post-anaesthetic tray.

Post-anaesthetic trays are often prepared as pre-packed trays in Central Sterile Supply Department.

FRACTURE AND DRY PLASTER BED

For fracture of spine, pelvis or lower limb

Additional requirements:

        Fracture boards.
        Roller towel and covered sandbags.
        Inside blanket.
        Cradle.

Method:

1. Place fracture boards under mattress to provide firm support and prevent sagging.
2. Make foundation of bed in usual way.

3. Place pillows, number depends on site of fracture.
4. Place roller towel over fractured part and fix with sandbags to prevent any movement of broken bone ends and further damage to soft tissues. (Omit if plaster has been applied.)
5. Cover patient with inside blanket and put cradle in position.
6. Place top bedclothes as usual, pleating over cradle to give neat appearance.

For wet plaster

Plaster dries by evaporation of moisture. Current of air is therefore necessary round plaster and patient requires turning at frequent intervals, *e.g.* 3 or 4 hourly. Length of time required for drying depends on size and thickness of plaster and temperature of atmosphere.

Additional requirements:

> Fracture boards.
> Inside blanket. Small blankets.
> Protected pillows.
> Socks.
> Perineal towel.

Method:

1. Place fracture boards under mattress to prevent sagging and possible cracking of plaster.
2. Make foundation of bed as usual.
3. Place pillows, number depends on position and extent of plaster.
4. Place protected pillow under limb where necessary.
5. Cover patient with inside blanket and small blankets where necessary, leaving plaster exposed. Put on perineal towel if required.
6. Place cradle over patient and make up bed in usual way, but turn back lower end of bedclothes to edge of cradle. Turn quilt under for neat appearance.

Heat should *not* be used to dry plaster, as: (*a*) steam generated may scald patient; (*b*) plaster tends to crack if dried too quickly. Discretion must be used if patient feels cold.

Care must be taken not to dent plaster by rough handling while still wet, as pressure will cause plaster sores.

DIVIDED BED

For patient with amputation of lower limb, to ensure stump is visible in case of haemorrhage and to avoid weight of bedclothes.

Additional requirements:
>2 sets of top bedclothes.
>Protective sheet and paper towel.
>Towel and covered sandbags.
>Bed elevator.
>Inside blanket.

Method:
1. Make foundation of bed as usual.
2. Wrap inside blanket loosely round patient, excluding stump.
3. Place bottom set of bedclothes in position over sound leg and under stump, well up into groin.
4. Place protective sheet and paper towel under stump.
5. Drape towel across stump and fix by sandbags to prevent involuntary movement, if desirable.
6. Place top set of bedclothes over patient so that end of stump is exposed.
7. Have bed elevator under bed in readiness for use if necessary, unless bed is mechanically adjustable.

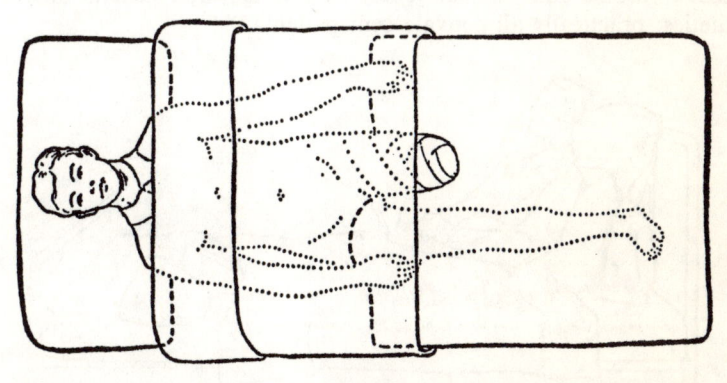

FIG. 6
Divided bed.

Divided bed also used for fractured femur with extension, omitting protective sheet and paper towel; towel and sandbags; second quilt.

POSITIONS USED IN NURSING

Recumbent
Patient lies flat in bed with one pillow under head.

Use.—To nurse patient at complete rest as it provides full relaxation; for examination of front of trunk.

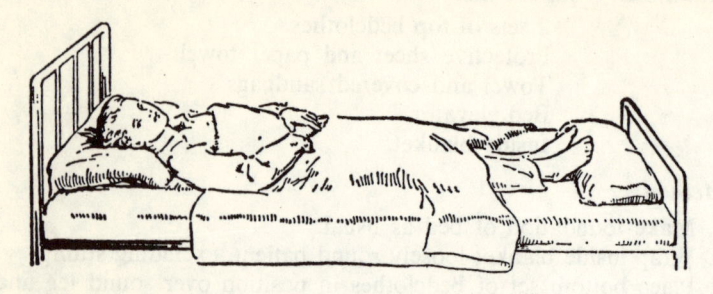

FIG. 7
Recumbent position.

Semi-recumbent

Patient is half propped up with several pillows, or reclining bedrest.

Use.—Widely used in medical and surgical nursing, *e.g.* gastric cases, chronic and subacute chest conditions; after general anaesthetics; practically all convalescent patients.

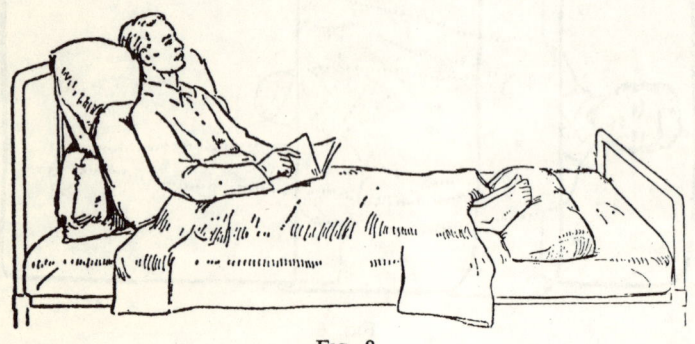

FIG. 8
Semi-recumbent position.

Prone

Patient lies flat on face, one pillow under head (which is turned to one side). Small pillow under ankles to prevent toes pressing on bed. Sometimes pillow under chest.

Use.—To relieve pressure on areas likely to become sore; drying plasters; nursing some types of fractured spines; burns of back.

BEDMAKING 39

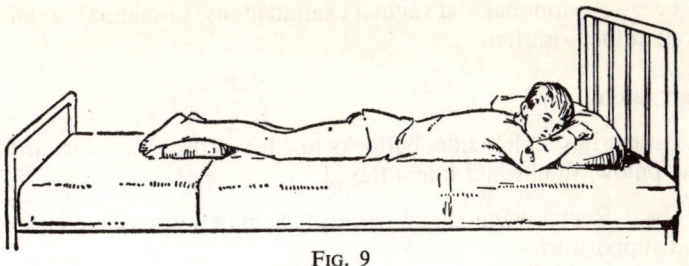

FIG. 9
Prone position.

Upright

Patient sits upright supported by pillows; may have heart table if dyspnoea relieved by leaning forward; may also require air ring.

Use.—For patients with chronic cardiac disease, dyspnoea or post-operative chest and heart conditions; for drainage of abdominal cavity.

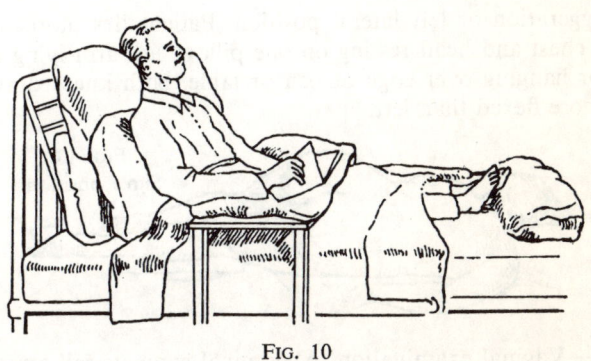

FIG. 10
Upright position.

Dorsal

Patient lies on back, one pillow under head; thighs flexed and knees abducted.

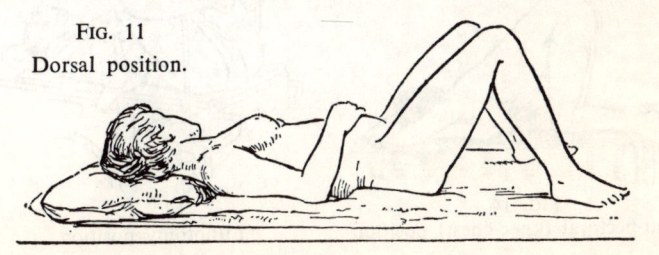

FIG. 11
Dorsal position.

Use.—Abdominal and vaginal examinations; bi-manual examination; catheterisation.

Left lateral

Patient lies on left side, buttocks to edge of bed, head forward on one pillow, thighs and knees flexed.

Use.—Rectal, vaginal and perineal examinations; giving enemata and suppositories.

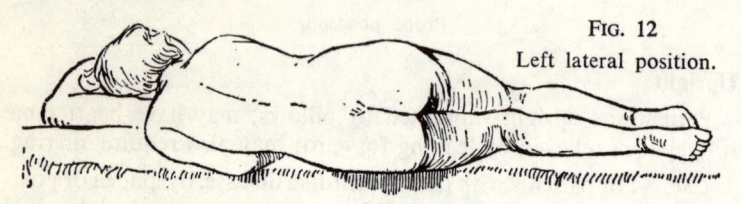

FIG. 12
Left lateral position.

Sim's

Exaggeration of left lateral position. Patient lies more towards prone, chest and head resting on one pillow, left arm lying behind back or hanging over edge of bed or table, both knees drawn up, right more flexed than left.

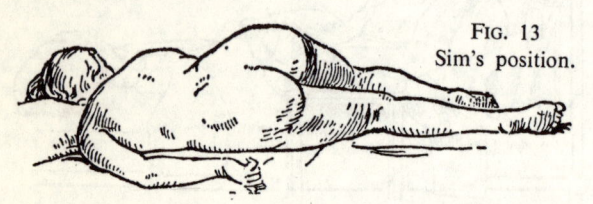

FIG. 13
Sim's position.

Use.—Vaginal examination. Abdominal contents fall away from pelvic viscera and vagina more easily fills with air allowing an excellent view of the cervix.

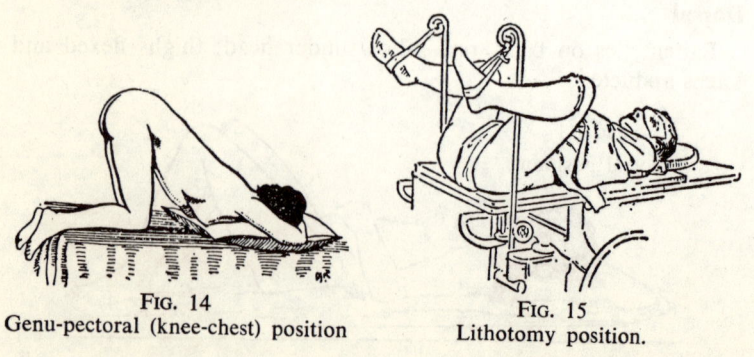

FIG. 14
Genu-pectoral (knee-chest) position

FIG. 15
Lithotomy position.

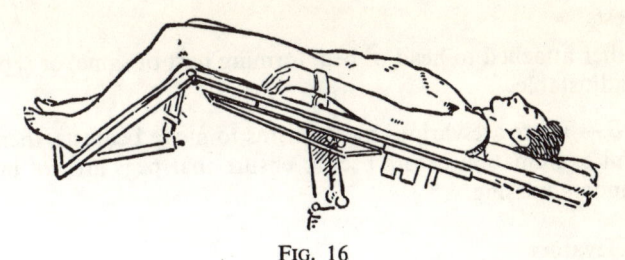

FIG. 16
Trendelenburg position.

Genu-pectoral (knee-chest)

Patient kneels on table near edge, thighs vertical, the chest rests on a small flat pillow and head lies just beyond, arms are flexed round head.

Use.—Vaginal examination; high colonic irrigation; in cases of visceroptosis to assist in replacing dropped organs.

Lithotomy. Trendelenburg

Positions used in theatre for gynaecological, rectal and other pelvic operations.

BED ACCESSORIES

Sandbags

Made of strong ticking of various shapes and sizes, covered by waterproof material such as plastic. Used for support and to maintain positions. Cover before use.

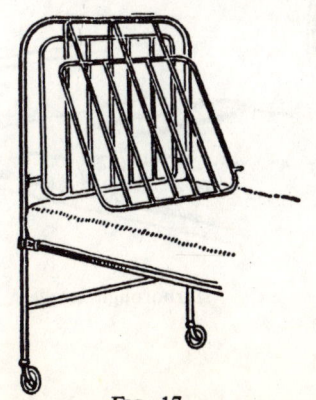

FIG. 17
Attached bedrest.

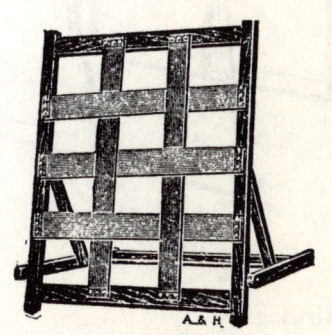

FIG. 18
Adjustable bedrest.

Bedrests

Either attached to head of bed, forming part of same, or separate and adjustable.

N.B.—There are various mechanisms to move bedrests, therefore careful examination before use, to ensure that pegs are not broken or winders missing.

Bed elevators

Used to raise head or foot of bed.

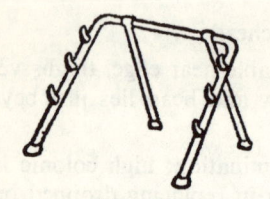

FIG. 19
Bed elevator.

N.B.—Many beds have attached mechanism for raising head or foot of bed.

Bed cradles

Made of wood or metal. Used to take weight of bedclothes from body or limbs.

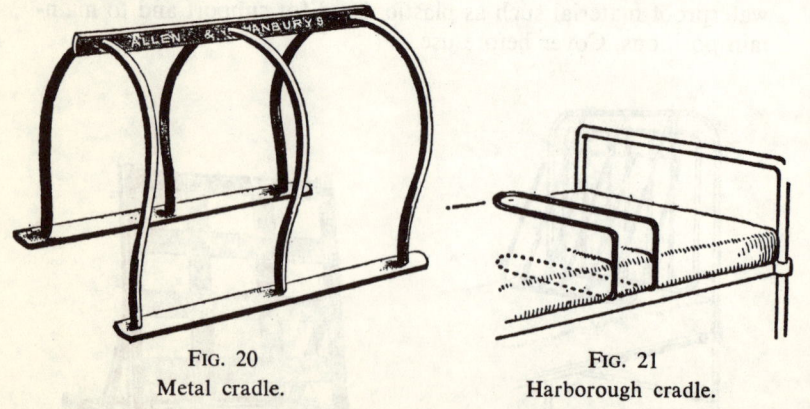

FIG. 20
Metal cradle.

FIG. 21
Harborough cradle.

Air-rings

Used to prevent pressure sores; must not be blown too hard, and should be covered before use.

BEDMAKING 43

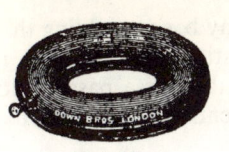

Fig. 22
Air-ring.

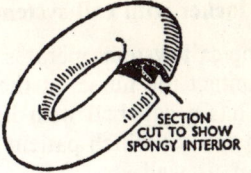

Fig. 23
Sorbo rubber ring.

Air beds, ripple bed

Filled with air, not too hard. Used for prevention of pressure sores, for emaciated and paralysed patients. Alternating Pressure Pads known as 'the ripple bed' which has alternately inflated and deflated sections controlled by an electric motor, which can control two mattresses, if necessary.

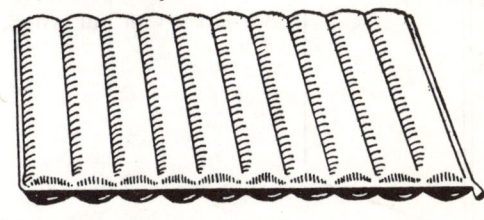

Fig. 24
Air bed.

Hot water bottles

Rubber; protect by flannel cover.

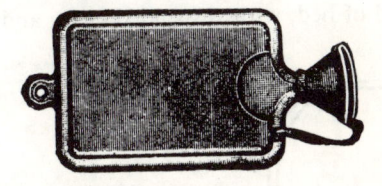

Fig. 25
Rubber bottle.

Fracture boards

Used under mattress to prevent sagging and to maintain even surface.

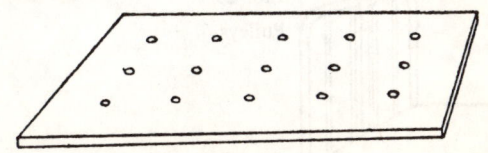

Fig. 26
Full-size perforated fracture board.

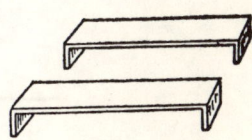

Fig. 27
Series of narrow boards to fit across wire mattress.

Bed locker with call system

The call system operates on a two-way basis, enabling the patient to contact the nurse, at the nursing station, and receive a reply. It also has a call bell with light so that the nurse passing down the ward can see which patient requires attention. There may be a radio socket as well.

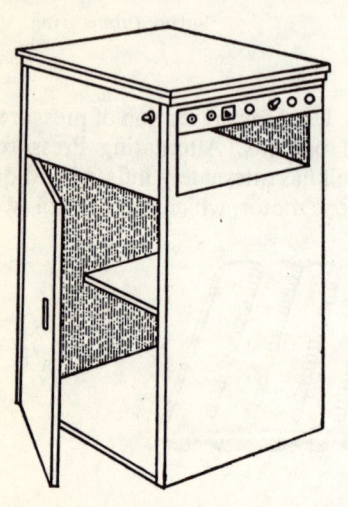

FIG. 28
Bed locker with call system.

Pulleys

Crooked bar over head of bed, with suspended chain and handle to aid patients in lifting.

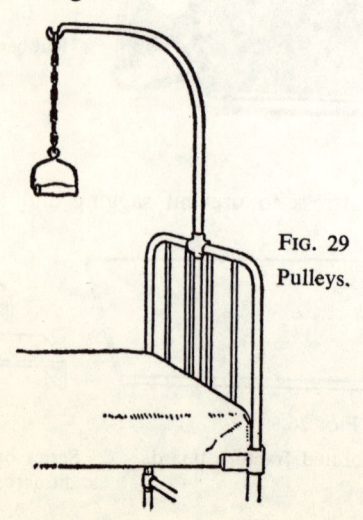

FIG. 29
Pulleys.

Bedpans

May be of porcelain, enamel, stainless steel, rubber or plastic.

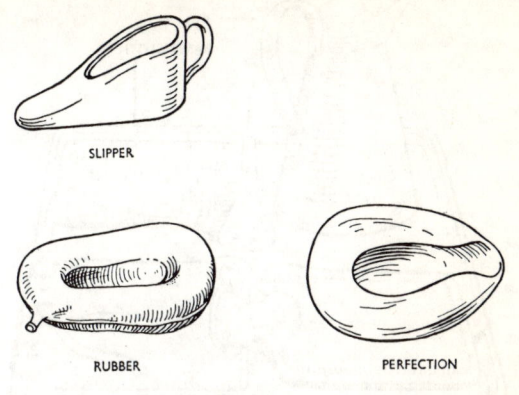

SLIPPER

RUBBER

PERFECTION

Fig. 30
Bedpans.

Urinals

May be of glass or plastic; special type used for female patients.

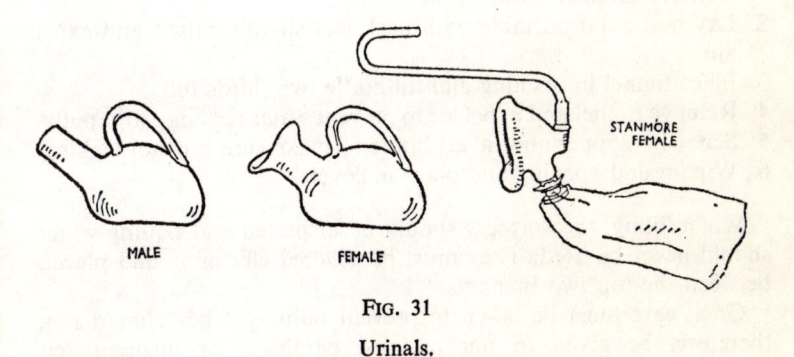

MALE

FEMALE

STANMORE
FEMALE

Fig. 31
Urinals.

CARE AND USE OF HOT WATER BOTTLES

Requirements on a tray:

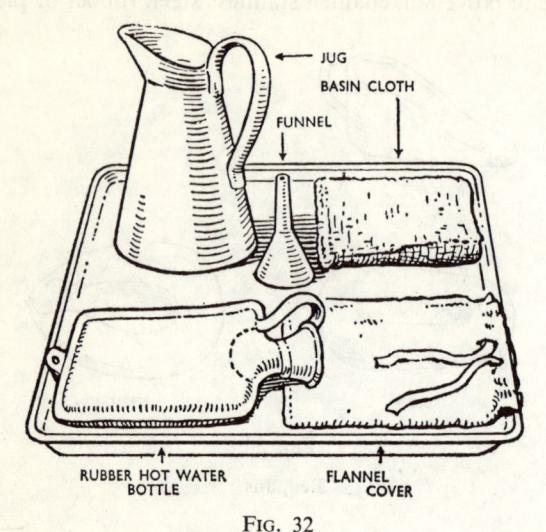

Fig. 32
Tray for filling hot water bottles.

Method of filling.—Rubber.
1. Remove stopper from bottle.
2. Lay bottle flat on table with neck end slightly raised and expel air.
3. Place funnel in opening and fill bottle two thirds full.
4. Remove funnel and expel air to prevent water cooling too rapidly.
5. Screw in stopper and invert bottle to make sure it is not leaking.
6. Wipe round opening and place in cover.

When filling, the washers should be inspected and boiling water should never be used. They must be covered efficiently and placed between the top two blankets.

Great care must be taken to prevent burning. They should not, therefore, be given to unconscious, paralysed or disorientated patients or those with impaired sensation.

After use empty and dry before storing.

If filling a large number, it is labour and time saving to collect them from the beds on a trolley, leaving the covers hanging over the ends of the beds, ready for replacement.

Chapter Four

GENERAL CARE OF PATIENT

Admission, discharge, last offices—Bed bathing—Bathing children and infants—Infant feeding—Prevention of bedsores—Care of mouth, teeth, hands, feet and hair—Giving and removing bedpans—Getting patient up—Care of the ambulant patient

ADMISSION

Patients admitted to hospital are either 'written for' from a waiting list or are emergencies.

Procedure

1. Patient is accompanied to the ward by a porter or receptionist, with notes and admission form obtained from a clerk in Outpatients or Admission Office, which is a section of the Records Department. Sister will have been notified.

   ADMISSION FORM RECORDS:
   (*a*) Name and address of patient.
   (*b*) Age and date of birth. Religion.
   (*c*) Sex. Single, married, widow or widower.
   (*d*) Admission and registration number.
   (*e*) Occupation or school.
   (*f*) Nearest relative for emergency. Telephone number.
   (*g*) Doctor recommending admission.
   (*h*) General practitioner (Home doctor).
   (*i*) Provisional diagnosis.
   (*j*) Date and time.

2. Welcomed by first nurse who sees patient or more often these days the Ward Clerk. Introduced to other patients and geography of ward.
3. Temperature, pulse and respiration taken and charted.
4. Written consent form for operation or treatment signed.
   (By relative if under eighteen years or unable to be done by patient.)
5. Weight measured and recorded in certain patients.
6. Specimen of urine obtained, tested and charted.
7. Toilet of patient carried out at Sister's discretion.

OBSERVATIONS TO BE MADE BY NURSE:
  (a) General reaction of patient, *e.g.* undue anxiety.
  (b) Cleanliness of clothes, skin, hair, mouth.
  (c) Abnormalities of skin and other structures.
  (d) Complaints, *e.g.* pain, breathlessness.
  (e) Last passing of urine, faeces, menstruation.
  (f) Medicines, etc., brought in by patient.
8. If relatives present, taken to see patient warm and comfortable to say 'Goodbye'. Given visiting cards and asked to furnish any information necessary regarding the patient, including, in case of infants and children, whether child is christened and wishes regarding christening if necessary; also full past medical history. Any questions should be tactfully referred to Sister.
9. All valuables and money taken home by relatives. If not possible, checked in presence of patient and sent to the treasury department for safe-keeping; receipt given when returned to patient or relatives.
10. Doctor sees patient to find out history of the case as soon as possible.
11. Many hospitals are now using identity wrist bands.

EMERGENCY ADMISSION.—When message received by ward, bed prepared as in Chapter 3. Appropriate needs prepared with bed when disorder indicated from staff in Accident Department.

DISCHARGE

1. Notify relatives and ascertain that patient has all necessary clothing.
2. Arrangements made for suitable transport. Rail travel can be arranged.
3. Social worker may need to check all is ready at home to receive patient, *e.g.* Home Help, supply of food, warm house.
4. Give written instructions regarding treatment to be carried out, and future attendance at the hospital.
5. Dressings or appliances should be freshly applied; generally seen by Sister.
6. Arrangements made for Home Nurse to visit if necessary. Small quantity of sterile dressing given, if patient is being discharged at weekend. Letter given from Ward Sister to Home Nurse giving instructions, if necessary.
7. Any observation or criticism of treatment, hospital, or belongings reported to Sister before patient leaves the ward.
8. Porter, ward messenger or receptionist accompanies patient to hospital door.

After discharge

Ward orderly or someone from Housekeeping department, sends linen and blankets to laundry. Mattress and pillows autoclaved unless they have washable covers. Bedstead washed. Locker scrubbed out and polished. Thermometer washed and lotion in holder changed. If separate toilet equipment used, a fresh set is provided from the Central Supply.

Notes—important that these are collected, the order checked and completed by medical staff and returned to Medical Records Department.

N.B.—Any equipment that is *not* expendable must be returned to C.S.S.D. If in doubt, ask. Most hospitals have losses due to confusion between disposable and non-disposable equipment.

LAST OFFICES

Performed for dying persons.

1. See that bed is adequately screened.
2. Comfort patient as much as possible, if conscious. Send for clergyman. Roman Catholic patients should have priest while still conscious, if possible. Remember that hearing is last sense to disappear and the patient may hear what is happening without being able to say or do anything in response.
3. If applicable, *e.g.* sudden collapse, resuscitation may be tried *i.e.* mouth to mouth respiration and/or cardiac massage.
4. When patient dies, leave relatives at bedside alone for few minutes, then take them out of ward. Comfort them and provide cups of tea.
   Note time of death.
5. Doctor must certify death.
6. Sister or Staff Nurse sees relatives, makes sure that they are fit to leave hospital and gives them written instructions as to when to return for certificate and belongings. Head Porter usually sees relatives to explain procedure with regard to registration of death.
7. Take notice of death to Matron and Records Office. Where Salmon Organisation, notice of death to Senior Nursing Officer.
8. Strip bed, but keep body covered with top sheet, remove pillows and accessories, take off personal bedwear, leave identity bracelet in position, if worn. Lay body straight, arms to sides and head on one pillow.
9. Place dentures in position and close jaws and eyes.

PRACTICAL NOTES ON NURSING PROCEDURES

Requirements on trolley:

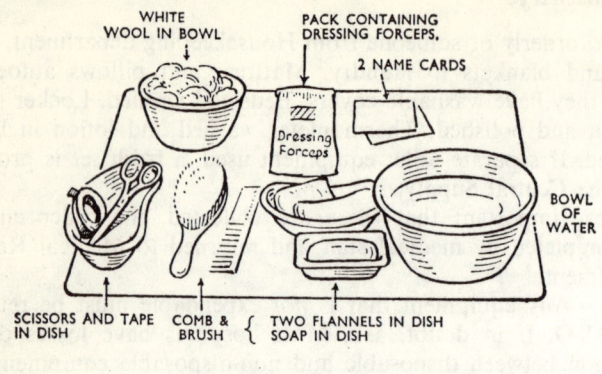

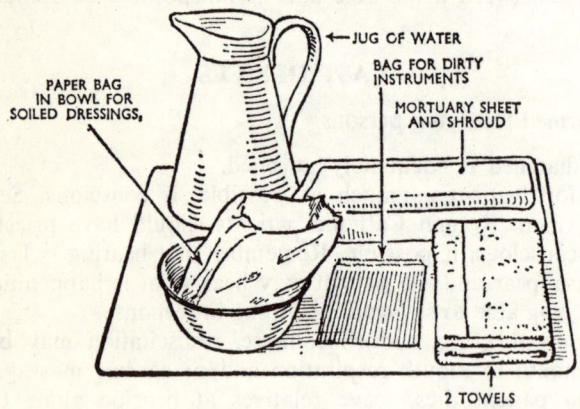

Fig. 33

Trolley for last offices to a dying person.

N.B.—Commercially pre-packed last office packs are now available.

Additional requirements.—Small tooth comb, dressings and strapping if necessary.

The subsequent attention to the body may be carried out in the mortuary.

Method:
1. Pack rectum (and vagina in female, if necessary) and nostrils (lightly, not altering shape) with white wool to prevent leakage and consequent soiling of shroud.
2. Shave male patient; if necessary.
3. Wash body all over with soap and water. This is not always

GENERAL CARE OF PATIENT

considered necessary, especially if the patient is cared for in hospital up to time of death.
4. Cut and clean finger and toe nails.
5. Put on mortuary gown (shroud).
6. Brush and comb hair: if long, plait in two plaits and tie with tape, otherwise arrange as worn in life.
7. Lay body straight with arms to sides and mouth and eyes closed.
8. Pin name card to gown.
9. Wrap body in sheet and pin second name card to it. Usually special instructions regarding type of pins used, if any. Particular method of using, so that mortuary attendant knows where to find them.
10. Ring for porter and trolley. Arrange screens suitably to make alley-way if necessary.

The procedure must be carried out quietly and reverently.

N.B.—If there are drainage tubes *in situ*, the wound should be adequately packed. Important to leave everything as it is if patient dies suddenly. Evidence required at post-mortem.

Bed and bedding dealt with as for discharge. Trolley cleared and locker turned out, patient's belongings listed, checked and packed ready for relatives to collect. Locker then scrubbed and polished. Bed remade and screens put away when everything returned to normal. This procedure is carried out by ward orderly as it is a domestic rather than a nursing duty.

BED BATHING

Requirements on trolley:

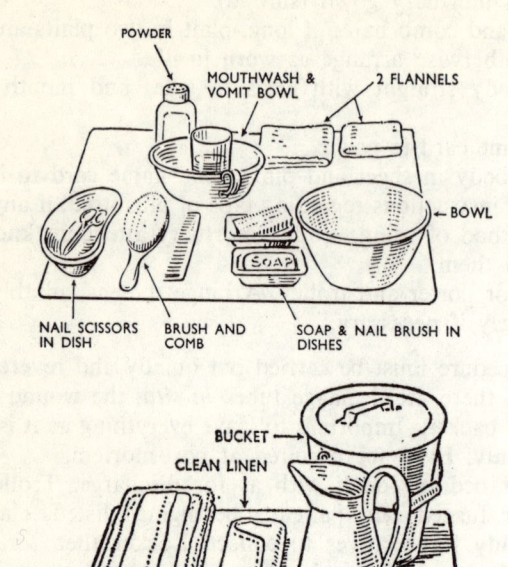

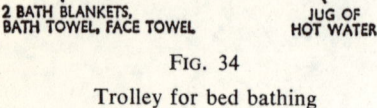

FIG. 34
Trolley for bed bathing

Stripper and laundry bag. Many of the items shown on trolley will be found in patient's locker.

Method:

1. Explain procedure to patient. Close nearby windows and screen bed. Give bedpan if necessary.
2. Strip bed, replacing top sheet or inside blanket, with bath blanket. Remove unnecessary pillows, but leaving patient in position which is best tolerated.
3. Remove cotton and plastic draw sheets and insert second bath blanket under patient.
4. Remove patient's bedwear and proceed as follows:

GENERAL CARE OF PATIENT

- (*a*) Face and ears; ask if patient likes soap on her face.
- (*b*) *Change flannel.* Top of chest and neck.
- (*c*) Arms and hands; rinse hands in bowl.
- (*d*) Front of trunk; take particular care under breasts and inside umbilicus. Change water, the genitalia are liable to infection from other parts of the body.
- (*e*) Wash between legs.
- (*f*) Legs and feet; rinse in bowl.
- (*g*) Turn patient on side, wash back and treat pressure areas. *N.B.*—Always enquire if patient is dry.
- (*h*) Roll bath blanket to centre, make foundation of bed (clean linen if necessary) and replace plastic and cotton draw sheets, rolling to centre.
- (*i*) Turn patient and remove bath blanket, make rest of bed foundation and replace plastic and cotton draw sheets.
- (*j*) Turn patient on to back, finish pressure areas, *e.g.* heels and elbows.
- (*k*) Put on patient's bedwear. Attend to nails.
- (*l*) Arrange hair and attend to mouth and teeth.

5. Shake and arrange pillows.
6. Make up rest of bed removing second bath blanket, leaving patient comfortable.
7. Put away toilet articles.
8. Open windows, remove trolley and screens.
9. Clear trolley.

BATHING CHILDREN AND INFANTS

In bathroom

Shut windows and collect requirements:

1. Child's bedwear. Dressing gown and slippers.
2. Soap and flannels.
3. Towels.
4. Brush and comb.

Run bath water, cold water first. T. 37·8° C (100° F).
Never leave child unattended in bathroom.

In bed

Give bed bath as for adult.

Baby bath

In hospital, infants under one year are usually nursed in cubicles.

54 PRACTICAL NOTES ON NURSING PROCEDURES

which are fitted with a bath or large sink. Nurse wears a gown, washes her hands and dons a plastic apron before starting.

Requirements on a trolley:

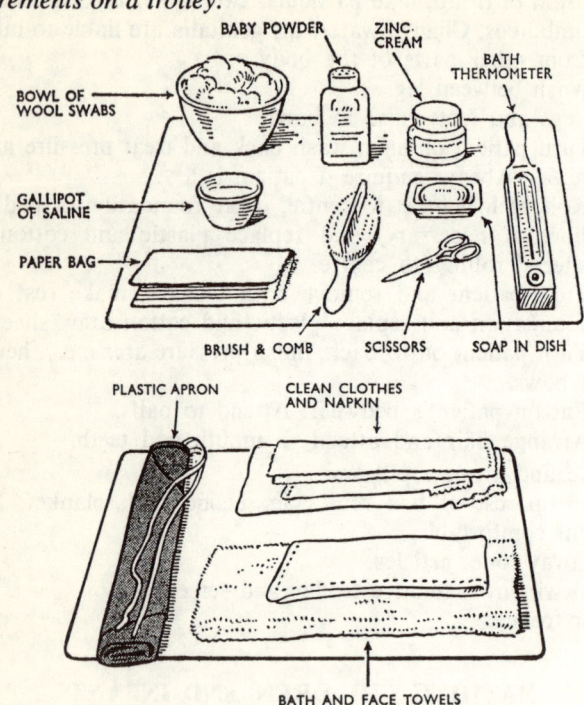

Fig. 35
Trolley for baby bath.

Two buckets, one for soiled napkins and one for soiled clothes. If no fixed bath, jugs of hot and cold water and a baby bath on a stool. Low chair. Screens. Temperature of water, 37·8° C (100° F).

Method:
1. Lift baby from cot and wrap in carrying blanket. Leave cot open to air.
2. Undress baby on knee covered by bath towel; discard clothes and napkin into appropriate buckets.
3. Wrap baby in towel, clean eyes with saline and wool swabs, using each swab once only and wiping from within outwards. Clean pinna and behind ears. Wash rest of face using wool swabs. Dry well.

GENERAL CARE OF PATIENT 55

4. Turn baby round and support head on left hand over bath, soap hair with right hand, rinse and dry.
5. Soap baby all over, especially in creases and between fingers and toes.
6. Holding baby securely with head supported on left arm, lower into bath and rinse using right hand. Rinse baby's hands first.
7. Lift baby out, dry well, powder if desired. Zinc cream may be applied to buttocks.
8. Dress baby. See that napkin pin is placed from right to left and not up and down.
9. Brush hair. Attend to nails.
10. Return baby to bed. Clear away equipment, and wash hands.

Infant feeding

Requirements on a tray:

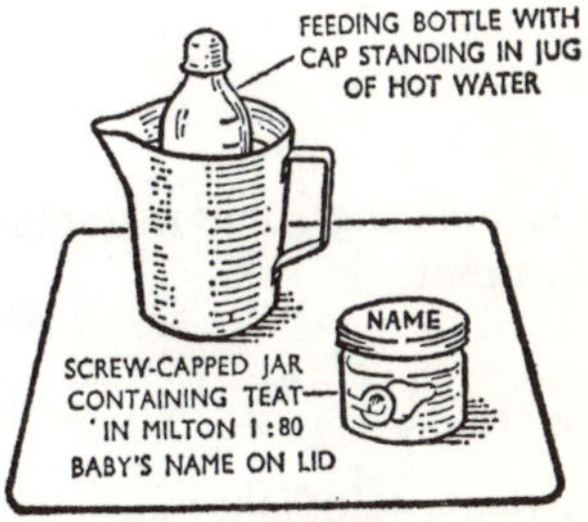

FIG. 36
Tray for infant feeding.

Method:
1. Wash hands—pour hot water into jug containing feeding bottle.
2. Don gown and change baby.
3. Wash hands and change plastic cap on bottle for baby's teat.
4. Pick up baby and, sitting on low chair, hold baby with head comfortably supported on left arm.
5. Feed baby making sure that teat remains full to prevent intake of air.
6. Allow baby to regurgitate wind in middle and at end of feed.
7. Replace baby in cot on right side.
8. Rinse bottle and plastic cap in cold water, wash with hot soapy water using brush, rinse and place in Milton 1 in 80.
   The teat is thoroughly rinsed and replaced in individual jar. Once daily the teat should be turned inside out and cleaned with salt before being replaced in Milton 1:80.
   Disposable bottles are now being used in some hospitals.

PREVENTION OF BEDSORES

A bedsore is an ulcer which is formed at any point where two skin surfaces lie together, or where pressure, friction or a moist condition is prolonged, as the result of confining a person to bed, when the vitality is lowered.

It may start as a crack or reddened area which whitens on pressure and remains white for some time. A white centre may arise in an inflamed area, painful at first, but not later as the tissues die and a slough forms, which separates to leave an ulcer.

Types of patients liable to bedsores

1. All acutely ill, especially if toxaemia is marked.
2. Helpless and unconscious.
3. Paralysed.
4. Incontinent.
5. Emaciated.
6. Oedematous.
7. Any patient who is suffering some metabolic disorder or whose blood chemistry is upset.

Pressure areas

1. Back of head, particularly in children.
2. Elbows.
3. Shoulders.
4. Vertebral spines.
5. Sacral area.
6. Hips.
7. Top of knees.
8. Ankles.
9. Heels.
10. Tops of toes.

Routine preventive treatment (must be carried out conscientiously)

1. Inspect all pressure areas at least twice a day.
2. Change position as often as possible:
    (*a*) Encourage patient to move about.
    (*b*) Turn helpless patient frequently—maybe every hour.
3. Keep bed free from irritating elements.
    (*a*) Careful bedmaking—no wrinkles, no crumbs.
    (*b*) No chipped bedpans. Careful giving and removing.

GENERAL CARE OF PATIENT

    (c) No long finger nails or jewellery worn by nurse.
4. Keep skin dry and free of discharges or excretions, which may cause chafing.
5. Use air-rings, air pillows, sorbo mattresses, wool ring-pads and cradles, alternating pressure pad or 'ripple bed'.
6. Promote circulation by massage.

Frequency of treatment

For helpless patients, *two hourly*, when turned or after bedpan.
For those with limited movement, *four hourly*.
For other patients, *twice daily*.

Requirements on a trolley:

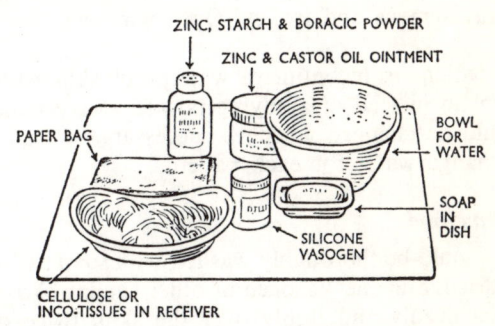

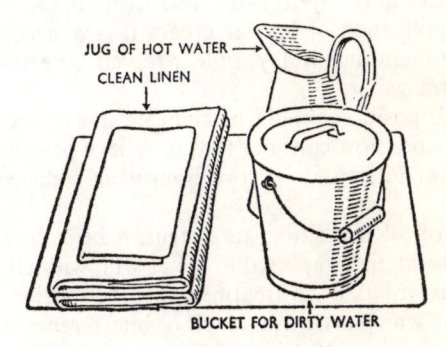

FIG. 37

Trolley for prevention of bed sores

Patient's bath towel and back flannel.
Stripper and laundry bag.

Method:
1. Explain procedure to patient, screen bed and close windows.
2. Strip bed. (If only sacral area to be treated, bedclothes may be turned back and part exposed.)
3. Expose area, protect bed with bath towel. Clean area with cellulose if necessary.
4. Wash area well with soap and water, using back flannel and rinse. Dry well.
5. Dust with powder to ensure dryness and to give a smooth feeling and make skin more absorbent.
6. Change patient's position and relieve any pressure by use of pads or pillows.
7. Straighten bottom bedclothes, remake bed and leave patient comfortable.
8. Clear away screens and trolley. Open windows.

N.B.—If patient is incontinent, waterproof skin with zinc and castor oil cream instead of applying powder. Very important that patient should be changed whenever necessary.

Always change water for each patient.

Alternative method:

The area should be thoroughly washed with soap and water, well rinsed and dried. Silicone Vasogen or other similar barrier cream is then smeared evenly and thinly over the skin, twice daily for 1 week, then once daily. Sprays are also available.

After the application of barrier cream it is unnecessary to wash the area more than once a day, unless fouled by excreta, and then only with warm water.

The patient's position should be changed five or six times daily.

Some authorities now consider that to relieve pressure on any one area at frequent intervals, *e.g.* two-hourly, is sufficient to prevent bedsores.

If, in spite of all preventive treatment, a bedsore does develop, the fact must be at once reported to Sister who will tell the doctor in charge, and his orders as to treatment will be carried out. *Trophic sores* are ulcers which arise as a result of interference with the nerve supply. They start suddenly as a blister or purple patch, which rapidly increases in size and forms a slough. Report any change in condition of pressure areas to Sister.

CARE OF MOUTH AND TEETH

General care includes:

1. Teeth cleaning twice a day, warm or cold water and toothpaste or mouthwashes as desired by patient.
2. Visit to the dentist twice a year, for routine examination. Any other time as necessary, *e.g.* toothache.

DENTURES.—Scrub with soap and water; rinse under running water. Give patient mouthwash before replacing dentures. If not being used, keep in water or mild antiseptic.

Special care for ill patients

Method:

1. Explain procedure to patient. Screen bed.
2. Place face towel under chin.
3. Remove dentures, if any; place in mug. Inspect mouth, using a torch.
4. Wrap gauze swab round clip forceps and dip into sodium bicarbonate solution which loosens mucus. Clean mouth (inside cheeks, both sides of gums, roof of mouth, under tongue, top of tongue) using as many gauze swabs as necessary and removing soiled swabs with dissecting forceps. Wooden applicator and wool swabs may be used to clean between the teeth.
5. Give mouthwash or swab mouth out with glycothymoline, according to patient's condition.
6. Finally, if lips are cracked and dry, white vaseline may be applied.
7. Scrub dentures, rinse and replace teeth, if condition of mouth allows.
8. Clean and reset tray. Remove screens.

N.B.—Use feeding cup for mouthwash if patient is lying flat. Babies' mouths do not require cleaning except in special circumstances.

FREQUENCY.—Two hourly, before and after milk feeds, or at Sister's discretion.

Requirements on a tray:

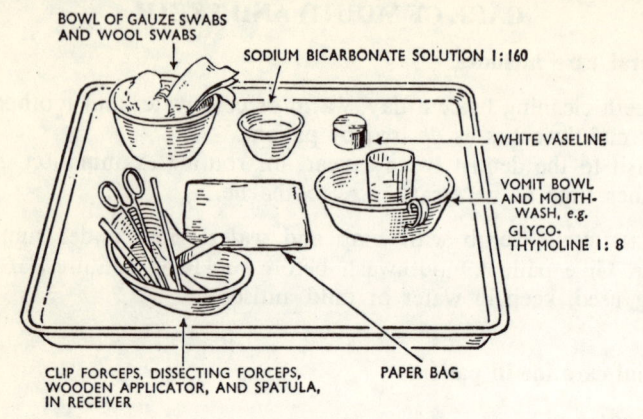

FIG. 38
Tray for care of mouth and teeth.

Patient's face towel. Mug containing water, if patient has dentures.

REASON FOR TREATMENT.—To cleanse mouth and promote normal flow when patient:

1. Is having nothing by mouth.
2. Has disease of tongue or mouth.
3. Is on a milk diet.
4. Is unconscious or unable to clean own teeth.
5. Has dryness of mouth with high temperature.

RESULT OF NEGLECT

1. Discomfort, sore lips, herpes.
2. Anorexia, halitosis, dental caries.
3. Parotitis.
4. Tonsillitis, adenitis, otitis media.
5. Gastritis, gastric ulcers.
6. Aspiration pneumonia, lung abscess.
7. Bacterial endocarditis.

CARE OF HANDS AND FEET

Hands

Must be kept clean; may be soaked in warm soapy water if very grimy, nails gently scrubbed; washed after toilet. When drying, cuticles should be gently pushed back and nails cleaned with an orange stick; nails should be cut or filed to the shape of the fingers.

NURSES.—Hand lotions and creams should be used. No coloured nails on duty. Neglect leads to 'hang nail' which may become infected and a septic finger result.

Feet

Washed daily; dried well between toes. If hard skin present, soak in warm soapy water and then remove. Pumice stone may be helpful in removing hard skin. Nails must be cut straight across to prevent ingrowing. Corns should receive attention. Chiropodist may be required to give attention, can be recommended by doctor.

NURSES.—Stockings or tights changed daily. Shoes should be well-fitting with suitable heels, having a broad base.

CARE OF HEAD AND HAIR

General care includes regular twice daily brushing and combing, to keep hair free from dust and tangles and to promote a good supply of blood to the scalp. Washing every one or two weeks according to type of hair and living conditions.

In bed, long hair is most comfortable in two plaits.

Dry shampoo may be useful for some types of patients.

In large hospitals, hair-dressing service may be available for patients.

On admission, head should be fine-tooth combed, at Sister's discretion.

Method:
1. Explain procedure to patient. Screen bed.
2. Place cape round shoulders and over pillows.
3. Remove ribbons, grips, etc., and comb carefully to remove tangles.
4. Take tooth comb in one hand and wool swab in other and starting at top of head comb down to end of hair turning comb up and ending in wool swab, wipe and examine for lice. Repeat process all over head, taking especial care, behind ears, nape of neck, crown of head and along hair line of forehead.
5. If not infested, brush and comb hair and arrange to patient's liking.

Requirements on a tray:

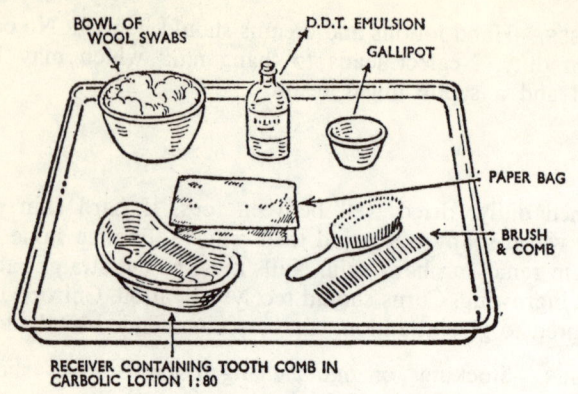

FIG. 39
Tray for care of head and hair.

Shoulder cape.

6. If infested, pour approximately one tablespoonful of DDT emulsion into gallipot. Parting hair, apply on wool swabs to scalp. Massage in with finger tips.
7. Comb and arrange hair to patient's liking.
8. Clear away tray. Boil tooth comb after cleaning. Remove screens.

In case of infestation, the head may be washed after twelve hours. DDT is insoluble in water and remains active for fourteen days if rubbed efficiently into the scalp.

Children's heads are combed daily and condition of hair recorded in the book provided.

Other indications for inspection

1. Regularly at Sister's discretion.
2. Spontaneously when a patient is found to be verminous.
3. Before transfer.
4. Follow-up treatment after a verminous patient.

WASHING PATIENT'S HEAD IN BED

The hair may be washed on the following occasions:

1. When a patient has been in bed for several weeks.
2. Before transfer to a convalescent home or another hospital.
3. As part of the treatment of a verminous head.
4. Before special operations, *e.g.* mastoidectomy.

GENERAL CARE OF PATIENT

5. On admission, if very dirty, and patient's condition allows.

When not possible to wash the hair at a handbasin it must be done in bed.

Requirements on a trolley:

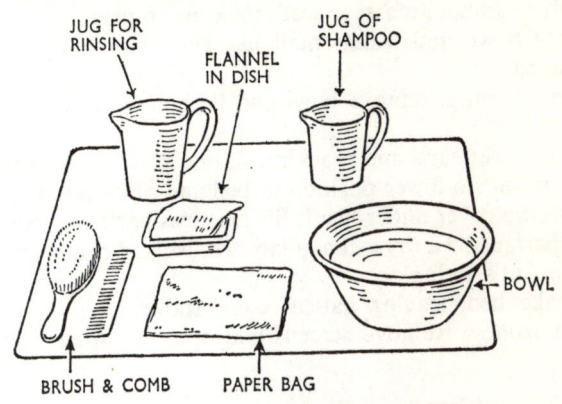

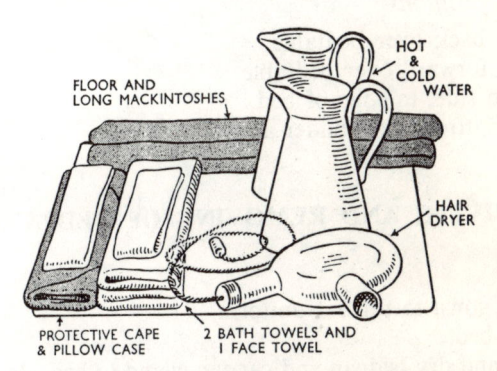

FIG. 40
Trolley for washing patients' head in bed.

Stripper and two buckets.

Method, carried out by two nurses:
1. Explain procedure to patient. Screen bed and shut windows.
2. Strip bed leaving patient covered by a blanket.
3. Turn down top of nightdress and put one bath towel round shoulders covered by the protective cape.
4. Brush and comb hair.

5. Pull mattress down bed, leaving enough wire spring exposed at head of bed to take bowl. Remove pillows and protect head of mattress and wire spring with mackintosh, place bowl in position. Lift patient up bed so that the head can be supported over the bowl. Give patient face towel to protect eyes.
6. Place water in bowl, and wet hair using flannel.
7. Apply shampoo, massage well, rinse and repeat.
8. Empty bowl, and using small jug, rinse hair until all soap is removed.
9. Squeeze gently, remove bowl and tie hair up in towel, turbanwise.
10. Remove wet cape and mackintosh and place in bucket.
11. Lift patient to lower position in bed and place pillow protected by plastic cover under head; lift mattress back into position.
12. Dry hair, using a dryer if available, brush and comb and arrange to patient's liking.
13. Remake bed, leaving patient comfortable.
14. Clear trolley. Remove screens and open windows.

Alternative positions:
1. Leaning back over bedtable.
2. Leaning forward over bedtable.
3. Lying on side, to edge of bed.
4. If hair mattress, turn under at top.

GIVING AND REMOVING OF BEDPANS
Method:

1. Put on gown to protect uniform.
2. Screen bed.
3. Warm and dry bedpan and carry covered to bedside; also toilet roll or cellulose in receiver.
4. Place cover over foot-rail of bed; turn back bedclothes without exposing patient. Ask patient to bend knees and press heels into bed, at same time, place hand under sacrum and raise patient on to bedpan, first removing air-ring, if used, and seeing that personal garments are out of way. If patient is helpless, sufficient help must be available to lift patient on to bedpan.
5. See that bedpan is in correct position and patient is properly supported.
6. When patient has finished carefully remove bedpan, giving support and help to patient where necessary. Cover bedpan. Helpless patient will require attention to toilet by nurse; there-

fore, tray containing bowl of water, cellulose in receiver and second receiver are required.
7. Make patient comfortable and tidy bedclothes. Give patient bowl of water, soap and towel to wash hands.
8. Before emptying bedpan inspect contents and report abnormalities.
9. Remove gown and wash hands.
10. Remove screens from bed.

USE OF SANICHAIRS AND COMMODES

Sanichair

The patient is helped out of bed into the chair which may then be wheeled out to the lavatory and placed over the pan. After use the patient may require help with toilet before being wheeled back and helped into bed.

Commode

After adequate screening of bed, the patient is helped out on to the commode which has been placed beside the bed. A blanket is put over the patient's knees. Nurse should remain within hearing distance, as an ill patient may unfortunately fall off commode. Patient must also be told not to get himself off commode.

After use help may be required with toilet before getting patient back into bed. Two people may be needed.

The chamber is then emptied and replaced in position.

N.B.—In both cases the patient will need facilities for hand washing, if he has attended to his own toilet.

GETTING PATIENT UP

Requirements: Dressing gown and slippers.
Socks.
Coloured blanket.
Easy chair and footstool.

Method:
1. Put blanket over chair at side of bed.
2. Assist patient into her dressing gown, socks and slippers.
3. Place patient's legs over side of bed and help her to stand.
4. Support patient while she turns to sit into chair.
5. Place pillow comfortably behind her back and fold the blanket over her knees.

6. Move chair to desired position and place footstool where patient can use if necessary. Give patient something to do, *e.g.* book, knitting.

CARE OF THE AMBULANCE PATIENT

Early ambulation brings many problems. No longer does a patient lie in bed most of the day and use a bedpan, he now requires a comfortable chair and table as well, and a toilet. Moreover, he requires assistance in getting out of a high hospital bed to the chair, and in moving some of his things from the locker to table, as well as assistance in getting from the ward to the bathroom or toilet, usually some distance away. Often there is no space for the patient who is up, where he will be out of the way of trolleys and stretchers. Meals in a chair can be difficult, unless small cantilever type tables are available. Footstools may be needed for small people. Floors should not be slippery and lockers or wardrobes should be available for suitable clothing. Slipping pyjamas and dragging dressing gowns are a hindrance and a danger to walking.

Chapter Five

TEMPERATURE, PULSE AND RESPIRATION, BLOOD PRESSURE

Variations in health and disease—Rules for taking and recording

TEMPERATURE

Temperature is the degree of heat of a substance or body compared with a standard.

A thermometer is the instrument used, based on the principle that all matter expands on heating and contracts on cooling. The mercury in the thermometer expands readily with small changes of temperature and gives an easy level to read. There are fixed points on a thermometer scale, namely boiling and freezing points.

Fahrenheit B.P.=212°   Centigrade B.P.=100°
F.P.= 32°   F.P.= 0°

To convert Fahrenheit to Centigrade subtract 32, multiply by $\frac{5}{9}$.
To convert Centigrade to Fahrenheit multiply by $\frac{9}{5}$, **add 32**.

The *clinical* thermometer is used for recording body temperature and is made of thick-walled glass tubing with a fine bore. There is a constriction just above the bulb to prevent the mercury falling as it cools until shaken briskly. Graduated from 35° C to 44° C (95° to 111·2°F).

In health the human body maintains an almost constant temperature between 36·1° C (97° F) and 37·2° C (99° F) with an average normal of 36·9° C (98·4° F). Temporary rises caused by excessive exercise or external heat are soon adjusted.

There is a slight daily variation between morning and evening temperature, being higher at night than in the morning, due to increased muscular and metabolic activity occurring during the day.

In disease, bacterial infection increases the rate of metabolism, causing rise in temperature.

Term used to describe a rise in temperature is *pyrexia*.

Hyperpyrexia describes a temperature over 40·6° C (105° F). It is dangerous to the body cells. Above 43·3° C (110° F) life is not maintained.

Hypothermia describes an abnormally low temperature. It may occur in some elderly or very young patients, due to exposure or inactivity. It should be recorded rectally, using a special low reading thermometer.

Types of pyrexia

1. *Continuous fever.* Temperature remains high, varying not more than 1° C in a day.
2. *Remittent fever.* Temperature varies more than 1° C and does not reach normal within twenty-four hours.
3. *Intermittent fever.* Variation is between normal or subnormal up to high fever or hyperpyrexia every one, two or three days, regularly.
4. *Inverse temperature.* Temperature rises in morning and falls in evening, *e.g.* tuberculosis.

Termination of pyrexia

1. By *crisis*, a sudden drop to normal within twenty-four hours, accompanied by a corresponding drop in pulse and respiration rate.
2. By *lysis*, when there is a gradual drop to normal over two to ten days.

Rigor

A violent shivering attack due to sudden disturbance of heat regulating mechanism.

Three stages: 1. shivering—rise in temperature.
                2. hot stage.
                3. sweating—fall in temperature.

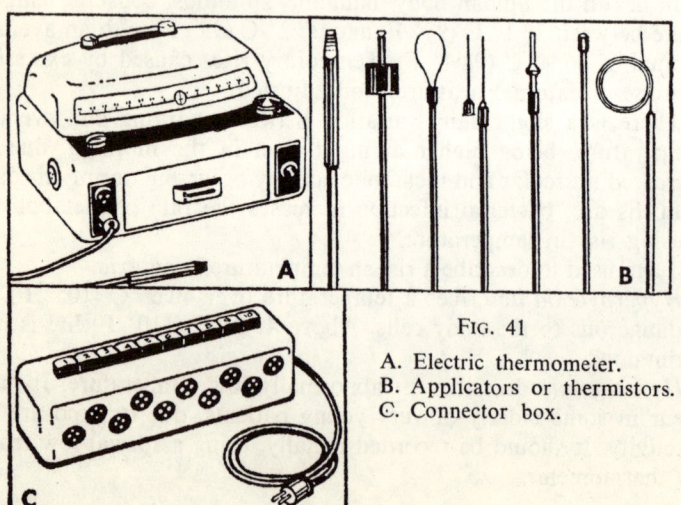

Fig. 41
A. Electric thermometer.
B. Applicators or thermistors.
C. Connector box.

TEMPERATURE, PULSE AND RESPIRATION

Sharp rise in temperature with no disproportionate rise in pulse shows good reaction on part of body against disease.

In any illness a sudden fall in temperature with no general improvement and high pulse rate is a serious sign.

Electric thermometers

These may be used for continuous recording of body temperature.

The essential parts being an applicator or thermistor, connector box and temperature scale. The temperature is recorded on the scale in one to two seconds after switching on the current.

PULSE

The pulse is a wave of expansion felt in an elastic artery. It corresponds with each heart beat.

It can be conveniently felt wherever a superficial artery passes over a bone, *e.g.* radial, temporal, posterior tibial.

In health the pulse rate is constant at rest but varies with the individual. Fifty to ninety beats per minute is usual with an average of seventy-two beats per minute.

Activity may double the rate, but this quickly returns to normal on resting. Emotion also increases the rate.

In conditions of decreased metabolism, the heart beats more slowly, *e.g.* complete rest or starvation.

Terms applied to the pulse rate in disease

1. *Tachycardia.* Rapid action of the heart.
2. *Bradycardia.* Slow action of the heart.
3. *Sinus arrhythmia.* Pulse quickens on inspiration and slows on expiration.
4. *Extra systole.* Extra beat followed by long pause.
5. *Auricular fibrillation.* Completely irregular pulse, very rapid and feeble. Auricle contracts 200–300 times per minute, all impulses not being transmitted to ventricles, which also contract rapidly and irregularly.

The apex beat must be taken in these cases as well as the pulse rate and charted in a different coloured ink on the chart.

When taking pulse rate note rhythm, volume, tension and regularity.

RESPIRATION

Respiration consists of inspiration, expiration and a pause. During the process an interchange of gases takes place in the lungs between the air and circulating blood.

Normal adult rate fifteen to twenty times per minute, increased during exercise or emotion.

Terms used to describe types of respiration

1. *Sighing* (air hunger). Long deep inspiration.
2. *Shallow.* Found in diseases of lungs.
3. *Stertorous.* Noisy, snoring inspiration.
4. *Stridor.* Noisy inspiration due to obstruction of upper air passages.
5. *Wheezing.* Sounds made during expiration.
6. *Apnoea.* Periodic cessation of respiration.
7. *Hyperpnoea.* Deep breathing.
8. *Dyspnoea.* Difficult or laboured breathing.
9. *Orthopnoea.* Difficulty in breathing unless in the upright position.
10. *Cheyne-Stokes' respiration.* A form of irregular but rhythmic breathing; there are alternating periods of hyperpnoea and apnoea.
11. *Asphyxia.* Condition when no oxygen can be delivered to the cells, *e.g.* drowning.

RULES FOR TAKING AND RECORDING

Individual thermometers usually kept in fixed receptacles beside the bed. Kleenex tissue may be used to wipe thermometer, then being disposed of into paper bag which is often attached to patient's locker. Fob watches are advocated for pulse taking, and ball point pens for entering the information acquired on to the patient's chart.

Temperature

1. Patient must be at rest.
2. No hot or cold drink given within five minutes of taking temperature.
3. Not taken immediately after a bath.
4. No smoking immediately before.
5. No talking while thermometer is in patient's mouth.
6. Thermometer must be shaken down. Wipe before insertion in

mouth, rectum or axilla. A special thermometer should be used for taking rectal temperature.
7. Dry skin if taking under axilla or in groin.
8. Leave in position for sufficient length of time, *e.g.* one minute.
9. Replace if thermometer has not registered.
10. Read immediately removed and record before thermometer is shaken down.

Pulse

1. Patient must be at rest.
2. Arm supported.
3. Get used to feel of pulse before starting to count.
4. Count for half a minute. If irregular, and in all patients with heart disease, always count for one minute.
5. Note down immediately.

Respiration

1. Patient must be at rest.
2. Patient should be unaware that respiration is being taken.
3. Feel, or watch, rise and fall of patient's chest.
4. Count for one minute.
5. Note down as soon as taken.

BLOOD PRESSURE

This is pressure which blood exerts on encircling walls of blood vessels.

Maintained by:
1. Strength of heart beat.
2. Tone of blood vessel walls.
3. Amount of fluid circulating.
4. Viscosity of blood.
5. Peripheral resistance.

Average systolic pressure is 120 mm. of mercury, when heart is contracting.

Average diastolic pressure is two thirds of systolic pressure, when heart is relaxing.

Factors causing rise in blood pressure:
1. Exercise and emotion.

72 PRACTICAL NOTES ON NURSING PROCEDURES

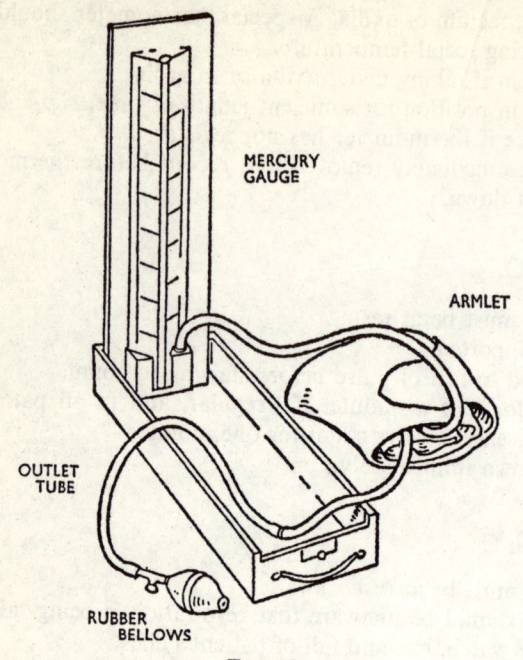

FIG. 42
Sphygmomanometer for measuring blood pressure.

2. Loss of elasticity of vessel walls.
3. Fever.
4. Chronic renal disease.

Factors causing fall in blood pressure:

1. Change of position, *e.g.* recumbent.
2. Sudden catastrophe, *e.g.* coronary thrombosis.
3. Excessive loss of fluid, *e.g.* haemorrhage, diarrhoea and vomiting.
4. Addison's disease.
5. Debility.

METHOD OF TAKING:

1. Explain procedure to patient, see that he is comfortably seated with arm supported and relaxed.
2. Empty cuff of air, pressing flat. Special armlets required for obese patient or the young child.
3. Place centre of cuff over brachial artery and wrap round arm, tucking in end neatly.

TEMPERATURE, PULSE AND RESPIRATION

4. Inflate cuff sufficiently to obliterate radial artery.
5. Slowly deflate cuff until pulse becomes just perceptible. Note height of mercury, which at this point is the systolic pressure.
6. Put on stethoscope locating brachial artery. Watch mercury.
7. Inflate cuff until pulse again disappears and apply stethoscope to brachial artery.
8. Release cuff until first regular beat is heard; note height of mercury which gives systolic pressure.
9. Continue to release cuff until quality of sound changes from a crisp lubb dubb to a less distinct blurred sound. At this point the diastolic pressure is read.
10. Write down reading as systolic pressure over diastolic pressure, $$e.g. \frac{120}{80} mm.$$
11. Remove cuff from patient's arm.
12. Make sure all air is expelled from cuff before rolling to replace in box.

Chapter Six

EXCRETA, URINE TESTING, ENEMATA

Observation and saving specimens of urine, faeces, sputum, vomit—Urine testing—Administration of fluids by rectum—Use of rectal tube—Fluid intake and output measurement.

COMPOSITION OF URINE

Normal

Fifty ounces daily; clear, amber, slightly acid, specific gravity 1010 to 1025, odour characteristic, containing:
water 96 per cent; urea 2 per cent; other solids—chiefly salts—2 per cent.

Sediment forms on standing and cooling; may be (1) urates (pinky); (2) phosphates.

Abnormal

1. Output. Polyuria=increased (as in sugar diabetes, larger water output to dilute sugar); oliguria=decreased. *anuria - no urine passed*
2. Colour. Smokey or red (local bleeding)=blood; brownish green =bile; blue=dye; bright orange=santonin (drug given in the treatment of worms); milky, opaque=pus.
3. Reaction. Alkaline=cystitis (inflammation of the bladder); does not necessarily indicate abnormality.
4. Specific gravity. High=glycosuria; low=kidney failure.
5. Sediment. May be pus, mucus, renal casts (lining of tubules).
6. Odour. Ammoniacal if decomposing; sweetish if acetone present; fishy if *Bacillus coli* present.
7. Contents. May be albumen, sugar, blood, pus, bile, etc.

MICTURITION

Simple reflex in infancy; voluntary with age.

Irritation of nerve endings in trigone by pressure of urine, transmits stimulus to micturition centre in lumbo-sacral region of spinal cord, from which passes the impulse to bladder wall causing it to contract, at the same time, the urethral sphincter relaxes and the contents are expelled via urethra.

DISTURBANCES OF MICTURITION

1. Retention of urine

Bladder unable to empty itself. Accumulation causes distension. If great, sphincter forced open leading to overflow, but bladder remains full. Retention of urine may be acute or chronic.

Causes:
1. Nervousness.
2. Atony: (*a*) disease; (*b*) pressure; (*c*) sudden release of pressure.
3. Urethral obstruction: (*a*) structure; (*b*) pressure.
4. Loss of nervous reflex: (*a*) spinal injury; (*b*) disease.
5. Unconsciousness.

Treatment is to remove the cause. If nervous:
1. Reassure the patient.
2. Apply heat to pubic region.
3. Warm bedpan; apply warm water to pubic region.
4. Run water within hearing of patient; wash hands.
5. Help patient to sit in as natural a position as possible.
6. Give hot citrous drinks, or Sodium bicarbonate, or Boracic crystals.
7. Catheterise, only on advice of Sister.

2. Incontinence of urine

Lack of control of act, in unconsciousness or paralysis.

3. Stress incontinence

Lack of control of act, during stress, *e.g.* cough. Reasons (*a*) prolapse; (*b*) old age.

Treatment for (2) *and* (3):
(*a*) Eliminate cause.
(*b*) Prevent bedsores.
(*c*) Prevent cystitis.
(*d*) Insert self-retaining catheter, release regularly; give daily bladder washouts, and change catheter frequently on medical advice.

4. Suppression of urine

Kidneys fail to secrete, so urine is not formed. Waste accumulates in blood and uraemia results.

Treatment. Medical.

5. Extravasation of urine

Urine passes into surrounding tissues, or may be intraperitoneal. Occurs in pelvic injuries and post-operatively on rare occasions.
Treatment. Surgical.

Examination of urine for diagnosis

1. *Admission specimen.* Clean vessel, soon as possible on admission.
2. *Morning specimen.* Before breakfast, clean vessel. If menstruating, wash genitalia, plug vagina and remove latter immediately the specimen is passed.
(1) and (2) are labelled in clean specimen glasses, tested in ward.
3. *24-hourly specimen.* Last specimen 8 a.m. thrown out. Then all urine saved up to and including 8 a.m. next day. Send whole or part to laboratory.
4. *Catheter specimen,* sterile procedure. Collect specimen by catheterisation into sterile container. Send to laboratory.
5. *Midstream specimen,* for this, the glans penis is thoroughly cleaned, the patient is asked to pass urine into a bowl and during the act the stream is intercepted by placing a sterile bottle in a suitable position to obtain a specimen.
This may also be obtained from a female patient, by first thoroughly washing and drying the external genitalia and then allowing her to pass urine into a sterile receptacle.

COMPOSITION OF FAECES

Normal

Four ounces passed once or twice a day, brown, soft and formed, with characteristic odour, composed of undigested and indigestible food, mucus, mucous membrane, bacteria (mostly dead) and water.

Abnormal

1. CONSISTENCY:
    (*a*) Constipated: hard, due to increased water absorption during long stay in bowel. (Scybala.) Common in elderly people.
    (*b*) Diarrhoea: frequent passage of loose stools due to irritation of nerve endings in intestinal wall; they pass through too quickly to allow water to be absorbed.

EXCRETA, URINE TESTING, ENEMATA

Causes.—(*a*) Aperients.
    (*b*) Bacterial infection.
    (*c*) Emotional states.

2. CHARACTERISTICS OF:
   (*a*) Rectal bleeding=bright red blood.
   (*b*) Gastric or duodenal ulcer=melaena. Dark, tarry stool. Blood has undergone changes in alimentary tract.
   (*c*) Iron or bismuth=black stool.
   (*d*) Obstructive jaundice=pale, bulky, greasy, offensive stools, due to lack of bile.
   (*e*) Undigested food in children=green stool.
   (*f*) Cholera='rice water' stool.
   (*g*) Typhoid='pea soup' stool.
   (*h*) Colon tumour=ribbon-like stool.
   (*i*) Intussusception='red currant jelly' stool.

3. SUBSTANCES:
   (*a*) Pus—burst pelvic abscess.
   (*b*) Gallstones—from bile duct.
   (*c*) Undigested food—milk curds, fat.
   (*d*) Parasites—worms.
   (*e*) Foreign bodies—buttons, etc.

To put up specimen of stools

1. FOR WARD EXAMINATION:
   (*a*) Remove toilet paper or cellulose from bedpan with sluice forceps.
   (*b*) Label with name, time and method of obtaining, *e.g.* by enema saponis.
   (*c*) Place bedpan in open-air cupboard, if possible.
   (*d*) Inform Sister as soon as possible.
   (*e*) Empty as soon as finished with.
   Baby's stool left in napkin, between two labelled receivers.

2. FOR PATHOLOGICAL EXAMINATION:
   (*a*) Patient told that specimen is required, so that she can empty bladder before being given a clean bedpan.
   Male patient is given urinal as well as bedpan.
   (*b*) Specimen taken with scoop attached to cork of clean specimen jar.
   Typical specimens of all parts of stool must be included.
   (*c*) If whole stool required, transferred and sent to laboratory.

N.B.—It is important that specimens should be sent to laboratory at once, with appropriate form.

SPUTUM

Sputum is material expelled from the respiratory tract, chiefly composed of mucus and inflammatory products.

It should be expectorated into a disposable carton, which should be handy on the locker.

Remove carton regularly and replace with clean one.

Measure contents if necessary.

Place container and contents in soiled dressing bin for incineration.

Observations

1. Amount.
2. Colour.
3. Consistency—watery or viscid.
4. Odour.
5. Frothy or not.

On standing, sputum may separate into three layers:
1. Deposit of green pus and tissue shreds.
2. Turbid brown-yellow layer.
3. Frothy top layer.

To obtain a specimen for bacteriological examination

1. Instruct the patient the night before.
2. On waking, ask him to expectorate into sterile sputum container, which should be covered.
3. Label and send to laboratory at once, with pathological form signed.

Any specimens sent by post must be packed in special containers and labelled 'Material for Clinical Investigation—Urgent'.

VOMIT

Vomiting is ejection of stomach contents by reversed peristalsis, when the muscular walls are irritated. It may be done (1) directly by means of salt and water, or (2) indirectly via the vomiting centre

EXCRETA, URINE TESTING, ENEMATA

in the medulla, which may be stimulated by, for example, a foul odour.

Observations

1. If preceded by retching or nausea.
2. Its relation to the taking of food.
3. If preceded by pain, relieved by the vomiting.
4. If regurgitant.
5. If projectile—forcibly ejected as in cerebral lesions, pyloric stenosis and intestinal obstruction.

Contents may be:

1. Food, partly digested.
2. Clear watery fluid, as in morning sickness or hysteria.
3. Yellow or green sticky fluid as in biliousness or after anaesthetic.
4. Blood (*a*) bright red, from nose and throat operations or severe haematemesis.
   (*b*) like coffee grounds, indicating a slow bleeding gastric ulcer.
5. 'Faecal' vomiting with foul odour as in intestinal obstruction.

Vomit should always be saved for inspection. Cover bowl, label and place in sluice. Report to Sister the amount and frequency of vomit. Empty and clean container immediately specimen has been seen.

URINE TESTING

1. Note colour and smell.
2. Take specific gravity. (Normal 1010–1025.)
3. Reaction. Blue litmus to red—acid; red litmus to blue—alkaline.

All urine must be acid before applying chemical tests.
If alkaline or neutral add one drop of acetic acid.

4. **Test for albumen**

   (*a*) Fill a test tube two-thirds full of urine, heat upper third. If cloud forms it may be due to albumen or phosphates. Phosphates disappear when acetic acid is added and urine reboiled. Albumen remains; *or* To 2 in of urine in a test tube add a few drops of 20

per cent solution of salicyl-sulphonic acid. Albumen present if turbid white appearance results.
(*b*) Albustix.

5. Test for sugar

(*a*) To 10 ml. (about 1 inch) of Benedict's Solution in a test tube, add eight drops of urine and boil. The result is recorded as blue, cloudy green, greenish yellow, orange and brick red.
(*b*) Clinitest.

6. Test for acetone

(*a*) To one-quarter of a test tube of urine add a few drops of 5 per cent solution of sodium nitro-prusside. Render alkaline by the addition of ammonia and saturate with ammonium sulphate crystals. A purple red colour which appears gradually and reaches a maximum in about fifteen minutes shows the presence of acetone or diacetic acid or both.
(*b*) Acetest.

7. Test for diacetic acid

To 10 ml of urine in a test tube, add 2 ml of ferric chloride solution. If diacetic acid is present, urine becomes deep claret. Diacetic acid, colour fades on boiling. If due to salicylic acid or aspirin it persists.

8. Test for blood

If there is no albumen present there is no need to test for blood.
(*a*) Pour 10 ml of urine into test tube. Add two drops of tincture of Guaiacum, shake, and mix. Add slowly a drachm of ozonic ether. Blood is present if a blue ring appears at the junction of the two fluids.

9. Test for pus

For a reliable test it is necessary to do this test in the laboratory.

10. Test for bile

FOR BILE PIGMENTS.—(*a*) To 5 ml of urine in a test tube add a few drops of tincture of iodine. Change of colour to green.
(*b*) Ictotest.

For Bile Salts.—Sprinkle a pinch of flowers of sulphur on surface of urine. The sulphur sinks into the liquid due to lowered surface tension.

For any Bile.—Shake urine in test tube. Froth becomes yellow.

11. Quantitative test for chloride

Measure ten drops of urine into test tube; add one drop of potassium chromate solution. Add one drop of silver nitrate solution at a time, shaking test tube after addition of each drop.

End-point.—Colour change from yellow to brown. Number of drops required to give end-point indicates concentration of chlorides expressed as sodium chloride per litre, *e.g.* 5 drops=5 g of sodium chloride per litre.

N.B.—Same pipette must be used throughout test and rinsed in distilled water after addition of each substance.

Clinitest Apparatus consists of a rack with test tubes and droppers, together with bottles of various reagents in tablet form with full instructions for use.

Phenistix is used for testing for phenylketonuria in babies.

Chemical Tests described above are rarely used nowadays.

ADMINISTRATION OF ENEMATA

An enema is an injection of fluid into the rectum, to be retained or returned.

Reasons for use:

1. To empty bowel of faeces.
2. To relieve abdominal distension due to flatus (wind).
3. As a means of applying local treatment.
4. To introduce fluids or drugs into the body.
5. For diagnostic purposes.

PRACTICAL NOTES ON NURSING PROCEDURES

Requirements on a tray placed on a trolley:

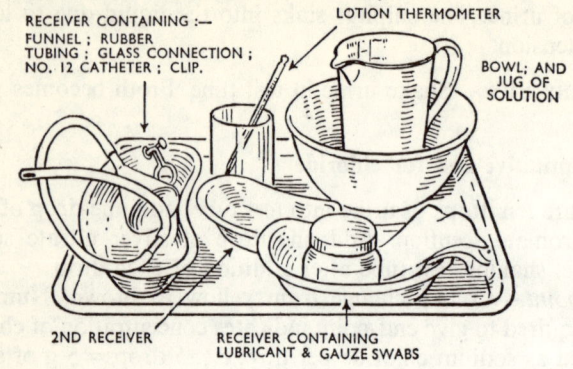

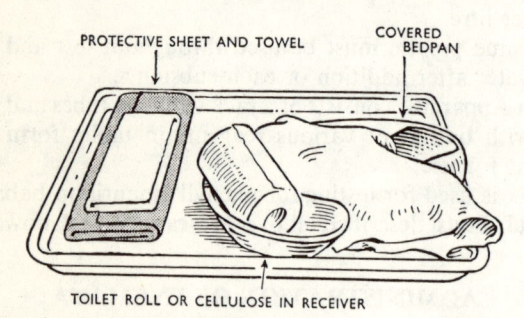

FIG. 43

Trays for administration of enemata.

N.B.—Disposable apparatus now mostly used.

Method:
1. Explain procedure to patient. Screen bed and shut windows if necessary.
2. Turn back bedclothes to pubic area and cover top of patient with blanket.
3. Turn patient into left lateral position and place protective sheet sheet and towel under buttocks.
4. Lubricate catheter and expel air from apparatus by running a small quantity of solution through, not allowing funnel to become empty, clip tube.
5. Insert catheter through anus into rectum, gently, for 3 to 4 in. Pour fluid through funnel, not allowing funnel to become completely empty until required amount is given.
6. Clip tube and remove catheter, disconnect from rest of apparatus and put in receiver provided.

7. Turn patient round and remove protective sheet and towel. Place patient on bedpan, propped well up if possible. Make sure patient is comfortable before leaving bedside.
8. Remove trolley and clear, cleaning apparatus under running water and running water through catheter from both ends; boil latter for five minutes, remove from steriliser and hang up to dry.
9. When ready, remove bedpan from patient; make patient comfortable.
10. Report on result; if necessary save for inspection. In certain cases note if flatus is passed.

Do not leave very ill patient or patient given enema for relief of flatus, while on bedpan.

Gown should be worn to protect uniform.

Complications

1. Faintness and collapse due to sudden distension of rectum with fluid.
2. Enema rash.

Disposable enema apparatus

Enema solutions and amounts

1. Simple enema. Use tap water, 1 to 2 pints; T. 37·8° C (100° F). Cleansing, *i.e.* evacuant.
2. Enema saponis (soap and water). Use soft soap (piece the size of a walnut or two ozs. of prepared solution) to 1 pint of water, T. 37·8° C (100° F). 1½ to 2 pints for an adult. 1½ fl. oz per year of age for children. Cleansing.

   To make concentrated soap solution:
   1¼ lb of soft soap to 8 pints of water.
   Use 2 oz of mixture to 1 pint of boiling water and add 1 pint of cold water to obtain 2 pints of solution at correct temperature.
3. Olive oil. Use pure olive oil, 4 to 10 oz, T. 37·2° C (99° F). May be ordered to soften faeces after operations on the rectum or perineum. Given slowly, retained for at least ½ hour (foot of bed may be elevated to assist this), followed by small enema saponis. Cleansing.
4. *Glycerine suppositories.* 30, 60 and 90 minims. Made of glycerine in a gelatine base. Cleansing.
5. Magnesium sulphate enema. Use magnesium sulphate crystals 1 oz dissolved in 4 oz of water (25 per cent solution). 4 to 6 oz usually given. Purgative.

6. Hypertonic saline enema. Use 3 drachms of salt to 1 pint of water. Anthelmintic, *i.e.* for the treatment of thread worms.
7. Normal saline. Use 1 drachm of salt to 1 pint of water. (1 or 2 oz of glucose may be added.) Stimulating or given to replace fluid loss.

THE USE OF A RECTAL TUBE

A rectal (or flatus) tube is passed to relieve abdominal distension.

Requirements on a tray:

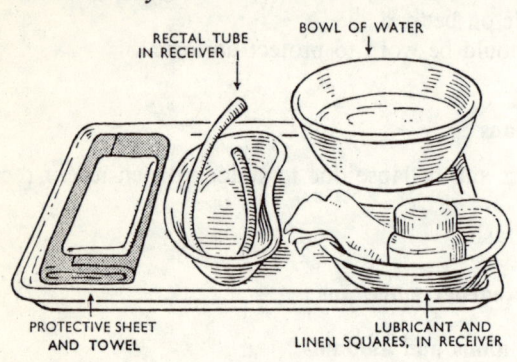

FIG. 44
Tray for rectal tube.

Method:
1. Explain procedure to patient and screen bed.
2. Turn back bedclothes to expose buttocks; place patient in left lateral position with buttocks to edge of bed if possible, and cover shoulders with blanket.
3. Place protective sheet and towel under buttocks, and bowl of water in convenient position, either on chair beside bed or on bed according to position of patient.
4. Lubricate rectal tube and, with distal end in bowl of water insert gently into rectum through anus for 3 to 4 in.
5. Leave in position for approximately 15 minutes. Bubbles will appear in water, if relief is obtained.
6. Remove tube.
7. Make patient comfortable and clear away tray and screens.

This procedure is rarely used nowadays, due to early ambulation of patient.

RETENTION ENEMA

Normal saline (approximately 1 drachm of salt to 1 pint of water) or tap water may be used by rectum to be retained:

1. To replace fluid loss due to:
   (a) Haemorrhage.
   (b) Vomiting.
   (c) Sweating.
   (d) Loss of body fluid as in burns.   T. 40·6° C (105° F)
2. To combat shock. T. 43·3° C (110° F).
3. To arrest rectal haemorrhage by its astringent effect. T. 46·1° C (115° F).
4. As a nutrient enema, with glucose added (1 oz of glucose to 1 pint of normal saline), when fluid cannot be taken by mouth. T. 40·6° C (105° F).

Requirements on a trolley:

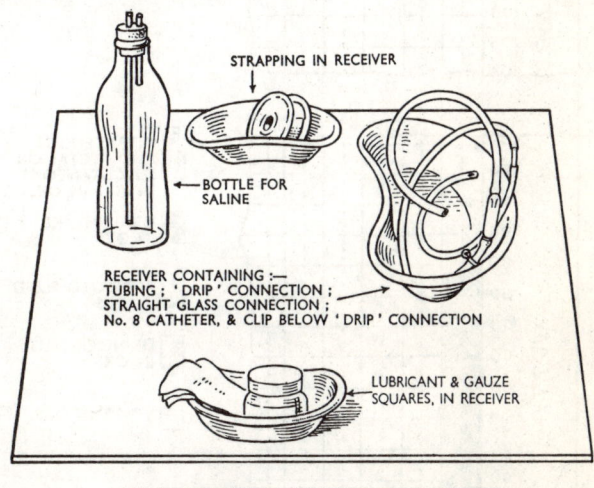

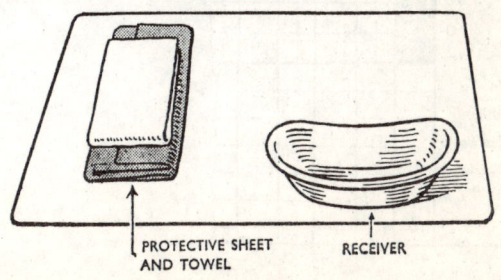

FIG. 45
Trolley for continuous retention enema.

Method:
1. Explain procedure to patient, making no suggestion that enema might be returned.
2. Make sure bladder and bowels are empty.
3. Flow regulated as ordered.
4. Raise foot of bed on bed elevator.

FLUID INTAKE AND OUTPUT MEASUREMENT

This is necessary to enable the doctor to maintain normal salt and

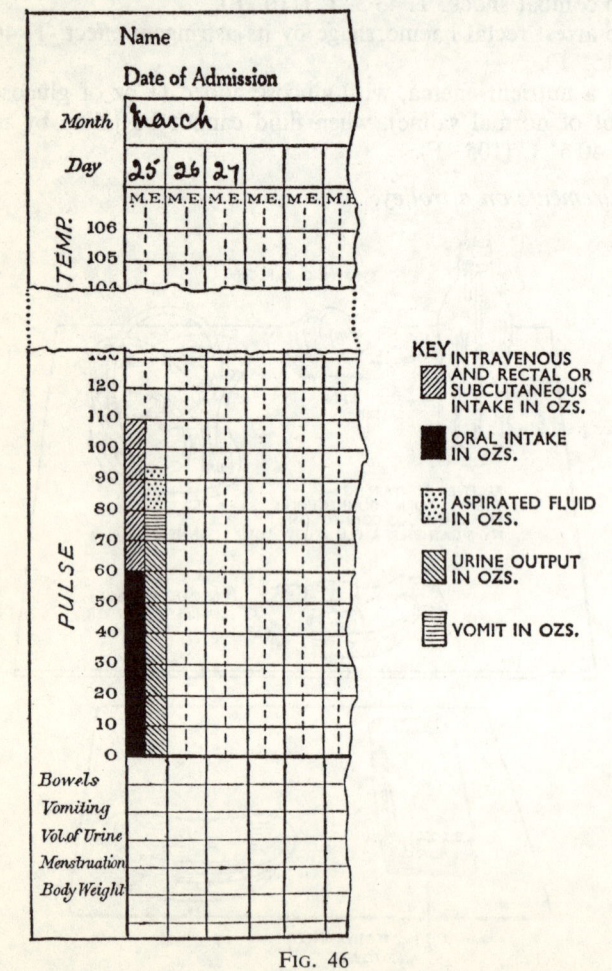

Fig. 46

Simple method of charting in take and output measurement, coloured crayon may be used instead of various black stipples.

water balance of the body in many medical and surgical conditions where food and fluid cannot be taken in the normal way.

All fluids introduced into the body, *i.e.* orally, rectally, intravenously and subcutaneously must be accurately measured and recorded on a special chart.

All fluids excreted from the body, *i.e.* urine, vomitus, aspirations and diarrhoea, must also be accurately measured and recorded on the chart.

Totals should be shown every 12 hours and allowance made for insensible loss, *e.g.* sweat, breathing.

Diagram illustrates suggested method of recording on pulse section of temperature chart, this shows at a glance the totals for 24 hours.

N.B.—A simple chart may be used to record the amount of urine that the patient passes each 24 hours. This may be all that is required. However, if more detail of intake and output is required most hospitals now have a separate 24 hour chart, for use.

Chapter Seven

INFECTION AND DISINFECTION. WARD DRESSINGS

Infection, sterilisation, disinfection—Central Sterile Supply Department—Ward dressing technique

INFECTION

Sources of infection

1. Human beings, *e.g.* person with an infectious disorder, incubating an infection or one who is apparently healthy, but disperses a dangerous organism, *e.g.* nasal disperser of the Staphylococcus aureus.
2. Animals, *e.g.* mice which contaminate foodstuffs, causing infections of the alimentary tract in human beings.

Spread of infection

1. Alimentary—by infected food and drink.
2. Contact—direct or indirect, *e.g.* contact with diseased tissue or handling of soiled dressings.
3. Airborne spread—by contaminated dust or droplet nuclei.
4. Certain insects—*e.g.* flies and mosquitoes.

Measures to prevent spread of infection

By Contact

1. Isolation nursing of the patient.
2. Care of health of all grades of hospital staff, *e.g.* reporting of colds and sore throats, septic fingers and gastro-intestinal disturbances immediately, immunisation.
3. Good facilities for personal hygiene, *e.g.* for hand washing and baths. In hospital arrangements can generally be made for non-resident nursing personnel to have baths if these facilities are not available in their place of residence.
4. Wearing of gowns.
5. Careful handling of soiled linen.

INFECTION AND DISINFECTION. WARD DRESSINGS

6. Proper diet to promote resistance to infection, and the hygienic preparation of food, especially baby feeds.
7. Individual thermometers and toys. Toys should be washable or destructible.
8. Aseptic methods when surgical dressings are carried out, including the use of a dressing station.
9. Disinfection and sterilisation of infected fomites.
10. Special measures to reduce dispersal or shedding of bacteria from the person, *e.g.* use of a nasal disinfection cream, or hexochlorophene dusting powder.

By Dust

1. Vacuum cleaners or damp sweeping and dusting.
2. Gentle handling of bedclothes; they must not touch the floor.
3. Covered containers for food and sterile articles; cupboards for crockery and cutlery.

By Droplets

1. Free ventilation and good natural lighting.
2. Bed spacing, *e.g.* 5 feet between beds or 8 feet between bed centres.
3. Care during talking, coughing and sneezing.
4. Wearing of masks.

Measures to prevent spread of infection by contaminated food or water, and by insects and vermin dealt with under Personal and Communal Health.

ISOLATION NURSING

1. Open windows as much as possible at all times.
2. Keep cubicle doors closed. Open swing doors with foot or elbow. Manipulate handles of ordinary lock doors by hand, regard outside handle as clean and inside handle as contaminated.
3. Place head of bed 18 ins. from wall.
4. Do not remove case papers and their holder from bed, or cubicle.
5. Work bare-armed.
6. Change uniform at once if it becomes soiled by discharge.
7. Wear a fresh gown to receive each new patient and retain for that patient. If not soiled, use admission blankets for patient's bed bath blankets. Keep in his locker.
8. Provide two gowns (one for nurse, one for doctor). Hang in patient's cubicle. If possible provide third gown for domestic

assistant. As gowns are worn to protect staff clothing from contamination, ouside of gown is regarded as contaminated and inside as clean; take care when removing gown, place on coat hanger and hang on peg to prevent contamination of clean inside. The word 'inside' may be embroidered on neck of gown as a reminder.
9. Nurse or doctor should don gown and wash and dry hands before she or he attends to patient, *e.g.* gives meal, changes napkin, handles bedpan, makes examination.
10. When attention to patient is complete, remove gown, place carefully on peg and wash hands well in soap and water.
11. Wash hands well immediately after touching patient, bed or any article used in his care.
12. Disposable crockery and cutlery is often used. If not, washing up machines often available, to which may be added a detergent such as Vantropol 1 ounce to 1 gallon of water. If neither available, crockery and cutlery must be kept separate, or be boiled after use.
13. Clean bedpans and urinals (after disinfection of excreta where necessary) in sluice room, taking care to avoid splashing. Disinfect articles by heat if possible, otherwise immerse in disinfectant, *e.g.* Izal 1 : 40 for two hours. This is only necessary if infection is in excreta.
14. Convalescent patients should not visit those on isolation nursing.
15. Equipment required for each patient:
Chair, locker, bedtable, 2 bath blankets, all toilet articles, washing bowl, jug and pail, thermometer and holder, pulse glass, back tray, mouth tray, large receiver. Crockery and cutlery tray, and if no facilities for boiling, means for washing and drying same. If necessary, equipment for dressings and treatment. Facilities for nurse and doctor to wash hands.

STERILISATION

Sterilisation

An absolute term meaning the complete destruction or removal of all living micro-organisms. This can be achieved by the following methods:

DRY HEAT.—In a heated cabinet at the following temperatures:
160° C for 45 minutes.
170° C for 18 minutes, Medical Research Council Memorandum 41, HMSO, 1962.
180° C for $7\frac{1}{2}$ minutes.

Infra-red, flaming and incineration are variations on the dry heat method. Infra-red is used as a method of heating a chamber to 180° C through which a conveyor belt passes, carrying the articles to be sterilised.

Moist Heat.—Applied as saturated steam in a chamber in which the pressure can be raised, (autoclave). An autoclave consists of a metal chamber surrounded by an outer jacket and lid. By means of a vacuum, air is withdrawn from the chamber and replaced by steam, the outlet tap is then closed and the pressure rises because there is no escape for the steam. This is a positive pressure (*i.e.* pressure above normal atmospheric pressure). The temperature and pressure can be varied to suit the nature of the article to be sterilised: *e.g.* rubber requires lower temperature. The average temperature employed is 121° C for 15 minutes.

Gamma Irradiation.—Cobalt 60 is used as a source of radiation in a chamber through which a conveyor belt passes carrying the articles to be sterilised. Used for some plastic syringes and intravenous cannulae. Exposure time varies, but equipment must receive 2·5 megarads.

Ethylene Oxide.—This is a gas used mixed with carbon dioxide or freon. The articles to be sterilised are placed in a chamber in which the gas is liberated (*e.g.* some types of syringe). It is explosive and toxic; therefore post-sterilisation aeration of articles essential.

DISINFECTION

Disinfection (Decontamination)

A term used to describe a partial process of killing bacteria. It generally means the destruction of vegetative organisms and some viruses, but not spores.

Methods: (*a*) Physical:

1. *Boiling in water.* Clean articles can be disinfected in 10 to 20 minutes. Some spores are known to survive this, so the method is not currently recommended for instruments.
2. *Sub-atmospheric autoclaving.* (Also called Pasteurisation as it is a variation of the original method devised by Louis Pasteur.) This can be achieved by water or steam at 80° C. Used for heat sensitive instruments, *e.g* endoscopes, and also for woollen blankets. It does not destroy spores unless formaldehyde is added.

(*b*) Chemical. Chemical disinfectants are designed to kill

bacteria, but may also cause tissue damage. Therefore skin contact should be avoided unless the agent is specifically designed for skin use. It is important that containers are kept clean and not 'topped up' without thorough cleaning and disinfection. Cork stoppers or cork liners should not be used, as the tannin in cork can inactivate some chemical disinfectants. Some plastic materials also inactivate them. For this reason, disinfectant solutions should not be mixed with other solutions (even detergents) and should be used at the *correct concentration for the correct immersion time*. Those in current use include:

1. *Alcohol.*—Ethyl, isopropyl or industrial methylated spirit. Used diluted with water to 70 per cent or added to other chemicals (*e.g.* Chlorhexidine). Used chiefly for cleansing the skin prior to injection.
2. *Aldehydes.*—formalin, formaldehyde, gluteraldehyde. Formalin is the solution made from the gas formaldehyde. It is used in vapour form for the disinfection of ventilators and incubators. Gluteraldehyde is used as a 2 per cent aqueous solution. Used for heat-sensitive instruments, *e.g.* endoscopes.
3. *Halogens*
    (a) *Hypochlorites.*—*e.g.* Milton, Eusol, Vim. The first two are used for disinfection of feeding equipment and in the dairy industry. When mixed with detergent *in a dry form e.g.* Vim, used for the cleaning of baths etc.
    (b) *Iodine.*—Used in aqueous and alcoholic solutions for skin disinfection.
    (c) *Povidone iodine.*—*e.g.* Betadine, Disadine. Used mixed with a detergent as a hand wash solution.
4. *Phenolics.*
    (a) *White fluids.*—*e.g.* Izal. Cheap and used for large scale disinfection.
    (b) *Clear soluble phenolics.*—*e.g.* Stericol, Hycolin, Sudol. Also popular for large scale disinfection and for reception of soiled instruments awaiting collection from C.S.S.D.
    (c) *Chloroxylenol.*—*e.g.* Dettol. Not currently recommended for hospital use as this is a weak disinfectant.

MISCELLANEOUS DISINFECTANTS IN COMMON USE:

Hexachlorophene.—Mixed with a detergent it is used as a hand wash solution, for skin preparation and can be added to bath water. It is especially active against staphylococci. Germicidal soap usually contains 2 per cent hexachlorophene, *e.g.* Cidal, Sterzac, Derl.

Chlorhexidine (Hibitane).—Used as an aqueous or alcoholic solu-

INFECTION AND DISINFECTION. WARD DRESSINGS

tion, *e.g.* instrument disinfection, skin disinfection prior to injection or surgery.

Savlon is chlorhexidine plus cetrimide (a detergent). Used for skin preparation and irrigation.

Quartenary ammonium chloride solutions, *e.g.* Roccal, Cetrimide. Have a limited disinfectant action. Used chiefly for cleansing dirty wounds.

There are many other disinfectants in common use in hospitals, but generally these are variations or mixtures of the above and are known by their trade names, *e.g.* Resiguard.

WARD DRESSING TECHNIQUE

A Central Sterile Supply Department is now available in a growing number of hospitals. Here all equipment for sterile procedures, *e.g.* dressings, lumbar punctures, injections, is cleaned with special apparatus, examined for efficiency, made into packs with disposable material and sterilised by steam under pressure or hot air in an Infra-red heated tunnel. The staff of the department issue the ward requirements daily, collecting in used equipment for cleaning, packing, and sterilising.

Non-touch method

Don mask and wash and dry hands. *N.B.* Masks are not universally used.

Mop trolley with Chlorhexidine 0·5 per cent in 70 per cent spirit. Dry with paper towel.

Method:
1. Explain to patient and screen bed.
2. Take trolley to bedside.
3. Adjust bedclothes carefully.
4. Wash and dry hands.
5. Tip pack out of bag on to trolley top. Open pack and tip instruments on to sterile field, adjust gallipot, pour out antiseptic.
6. Don polythene gloves or bags, remove soiled dressings and discard both into paper bag on bottom shelf. Carry out dressing, using forceps.
7. When dressing is completed, discard forceps into special bag. Fold down tops of bags and place in appropriate pedal bins.
8. Make patient comfortable.
9. Clear and reset trolley.

Requirements:

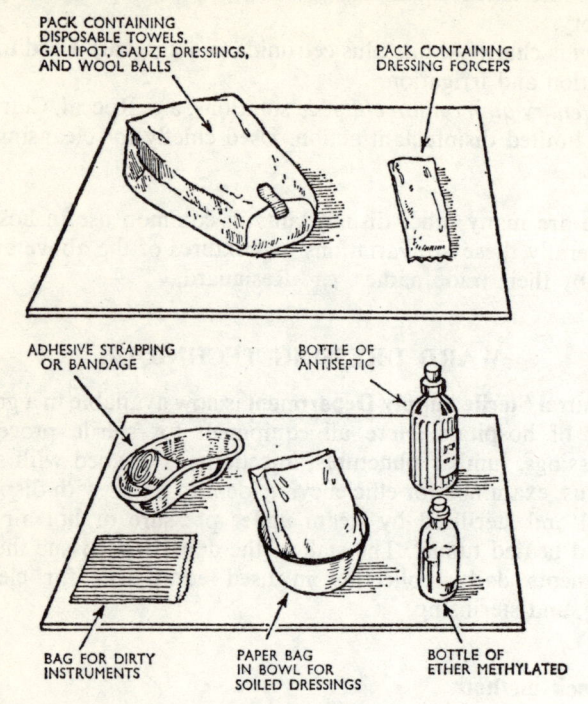

Fig. 47
Trolley for ward dressing.

Soiled instruments are returned to C.S.S.D. for cleaning, repacking and sterilising.

It is advisable that two nurses should do dressings together, if possible. When non-touch method is used it is unnecessary to subject the hands and arms to prolonged and frequent scrubbing, this only makes them sore and allows entry of pathogenic bacteria, which is positively dangerous.

N.B. Disposable masks should be discarded after 1 hour or after sneezing.

The use of polythene gloves when handling septic dressings is advocated. It is difficult to remove septic organisms from the hands by washing and it is far safer to prevent them getting on the skin at all.

Nobecutane spray is now used quite frequently for wounds. This provides an airtight, waterproof covering which protects the wound and requires no attention until clips or stitches are removed.

Chapter Eight

ADMINISTRATION OF MEDICINES

Weights and measures—Rules for administering medicines by mouth—Alternative routes—Hypodermic and intramuscular injections

WEIGHTS AND MEASURES

Imperial (English) and Metric Systems

1. IMPERIAL.—*Weight* (apothecaries') used in compounding medicines.

   60 grains = 1 drachm
   8 drachms = 1 ounce

   (avoirdupois) used for household substances.
   437·5 grains = 1 ounce
   16 ounces = 1 pound

   Volume (fluid).
   60 minims = 1 drachm
   8 drachms = 1 ounce (480 minims)
   20 ounces = 1 pint
   8 pints = 1 gallon

2. METRIC.—*Weight.*
   1,000 milligrammes = 1 gramme
   1,000 grammes = 1 kilogramme

   Volume.
   1,000 cubic centimetres = 1 litre
   1 cubic centimetre or millilitre = 1 ml

EQUIVALENT METRIC AND IMPERIAL MEASURES
WEIGHTS

2 lb. 3¼ oz.	1 kg	¾ gr	50 mg
1 oz	30 g	½ gr	30 mg
½ oz	15 g	⅓ gr	20 mg
120 gr	8 g	¼ gr	15 mg
60 gr	4 g	⅙ gr	10 mg
30 gr	2 g	⅛ gr	8 mg

15 gr	1 g (1,000 mg)	$\frac{1}{10}$ gr	6 mg
10 gr	600 mg	$\frac{1}{20}$ gr	3 mg
7½ gr	500 mg	$\frac{1}{60}$ gr	1 mg
5 gr	300 mg	$\frac{1}{100}$ gr	0·6 mg
4 gr	250 mg	$\frac{1}{120}$ gr	0·5 mg
3 gr	200 mg	$\frac{1}{200}$ gr	0·3 mg
2½ gr	100 mg	$\frac{1}{300}$ gr	0·2 mg
1 gr	60 mg	$\frac{1}{600}$ gr	0·1 mg

LIQUIDS

40 fluid ounces (1 quart)	1,200 ml	45 min	3·0 ml
35 fluid ounces	1,000 ml	30 min	2·0 ml
20 fluid ounces (1 pint)	568 ml	15 min	1·0 ml
17 fluid ounces	500 ml	12 min	0·75 ml
10 fluid ounces (½ pint)	284 ml	10 min	0·6 ml
3½ fluid ounces	100 ml	8 min	0·5 ml
1 fluid ounce	30 ml	5 min	0·3 ml
½ fluid ounce	15 ml	4 min	0·25 ml
2½ fluid drachms	10 ml	3 min	0·2 ml
1 fluid drachms (60 min)	4 ml	1½ min	0·1 ml

DOMESTIC MEASURES

```
            8 teaspoonfuls =1 ounce
                          =2 tablespoonfuls
                          =4 dessertspoonfuls
            1 teacupful   =5 ounces
            1 tumbler     =8 ounces
```

Percentage solutions

METRIC SYSTEM.—1 g is the weight of 1 ml (cc) of water (at 4° C). Therefore 1 g of drug dissolved in 100 ml (cc) or 100 g of water equals 1 per cent solution.

IMPERIAL SYSTEM (ENGLISH).—437·5 gr (1 ounce weight) is the weight of 480 minims of water (1 ounce volume). Therefore 100 gr is the weight of 110 minims of water.

$$\frac{480}{437 \cdot 5} \times 100$$

In this case a 1 per cent solution would be 1 gr of drug dissolved in 100 gr of water (110 minims).

To dilute stock solutions of lotions

$$\frac{\text{Strength of stock solution}}{\text{Strength of solution required}} \times \frac{\text{amount of solution required in}}{\text{ounces}}$$

$$= \frac{\text{number of ounces of stock solution to be added to}}{\text{water up to total amount of solution required:}}$$

e.g. 1 pint of 1:80 solution required from a stock solution 1:20.

$$\frac{\cancel{20}^{\ 1}}{\cancel{80}_{\ 4}^{\ 1}} \times \frac{\cancel{20}^{\ 5}}{1} = \left.\begin{array}{l}\text{5 ounces stock solution}\\ \text{15 ounces water}\end{array}\right\} \text{20 ounces 1:80}$$

To dilute potent drugs

$$\frac{\text{Strength wanted}}{\text{Strength available}} \times \text{number of minims known}$$

e.g. ⅛ gr. morphia from ¼ gr. in 24 minims

$$\frac{1}{8} \div \frac{1}{4} \times 24 = \frac{1}{\cancel{8}_{\ 1}} \times \frac{4}{1} \times \frac{\cancel{24}^{\ 3}}{1} = 12 \text{ minims.}$$

ADMINISTRATION OF MEDICINES

Storage of medicines and drugs

Precautionary measures are taken in hospital for the safe custody of medicines, drugs and lotions to prevent accidents occurring.

It is desirable that separate cupboards should be used and be kept locked:

1. Drugs and lotions for external use—these should be dispensed in distinctive bottles and be marked 'for external use only'.
2. Medicines and drugs for internal use, including drugs on Schedule 1 and 4 which are kept in a *special* poison cupboard.
3. Dangerous drugs which come under the Dangerous Drugs Act, *e.g.* habit forming drugs. This cupboard is kept locked at all times and the key carried by the nurse in charge.

Rules for administering medicines by mouth

1. Read label, before removing bottle from shelf, again before pouring out dose, check with patient's prescription sheet.
2. Shake bottle, holding cork, by inverting gently several times.
3. Hold bottle, label uppermost (soiled label is unsightly and dangerous because illegible), in right hand.
4. Remove cork with little finger of left hand.
5. Holding medicine glass in left hand, measure dose at eye level.
6. Check again with patient's prescription sheet before handing to patient.
7. Give at correct time and see that patient takes it.
8. If medicine contains sediment, stir immediately before patient drinks it.
9. Potent drugs *must* be checked by a trained nurse.
10. Once a dose of medicine is poured out it must never be returned to the bottle.
11. Never give medicines from unlabelled bottles or other containers.
12. Medicine glasses or measures may be disposable. If not they are collected into a bowl or on a tray, at the end of the round, and washed in the kitchen using hot water containing a detergent/sterilising agent, rinsed in hot clean water and dried.

Requirements on tray for one:

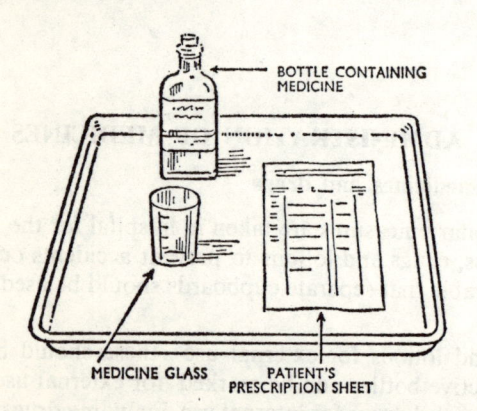

FIG. 48

Tray for administration of medicines.

ADMINISTRATION OF MEDICINES

Requirements on top shelf of trolley for large numbers:

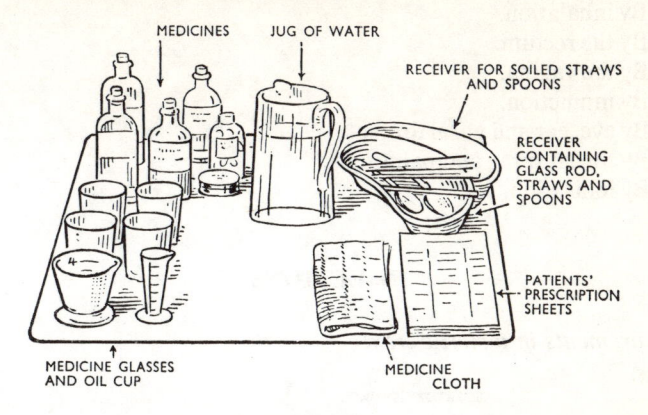

FIG. 49
Trolley for administration of medicines.

General remarks

1. Medicine containing iron stains the teeth. Use straw or give mouthwash after administration.
2. If unpleasant taste, give drink, fruit or sweet after dose if allowed. Holding nose may help.
3. Give powders by placing on tongue and follow with a drink.
4. Give pills and capsules with a drink.
5. Oily substances can be given in lemon or orange juice or beaten up in warm milk. Use china measure.

Disadvantages of medicine by mouth

1. Patient may not swallow medicine.
2. Medicine may only be partially absorbed, or destroyed by gastric juice.
3. Drug may irritate the alimentary tract causing vomiting and diarrhoea.

Alternative methods of introducing medicines into the body

1. Hypodermically
2. Intramuscularly
3. Intravenously } Parenterally
4. Intrathecally
5. Sublinqually

6. By implantation.
7. By inhalation.
8. By the rectum.
9. By the vagina.
10. By injunction.
11. By eye, ear and nasal drops.
12. By throat spray and painting.
13. By ionisation.

INJECTIONS

Requirements in a sterile tray:

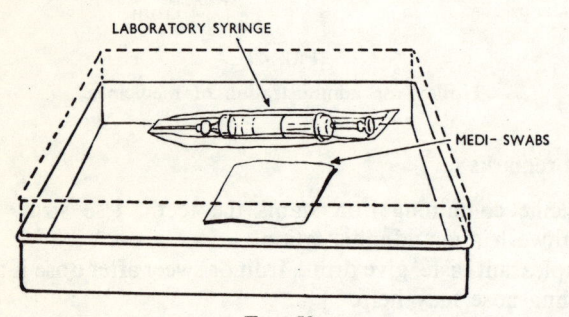

FIG. 50
Tray for injections.

Method for hypodermic injection:

1. Wash and dry hands.
2. File off top of ampoule and draw contents into syringe.
3. Expel air into a swab and check correct amount of drug to be given, with patient's prescription sheet. All drugs (both the amount and its administration) must be checked by a trained nurse.
4. Replace syringe on tray.
5. Carry to bedside. Inform patient. Expose area, *e.g.* upper arm.
6. Clean skin. Insert needle at slight angle, withdraw piston to ascertain not in blood vessel, push piston home, withdraw needle with swab applied to skin, massage to hasten absorption.
7. Leave patient comfortable.
8. Fill in drug book. Sign.
9. Rinse syringe and needle, unless disposable type has been used.

ADMINISTRATION OF MEDICINES 101

Fig. 51
Injections.

A = HYPODERMIC INJECTION
B = INTRAMUSCULAR INJECTION

Method for intramuscular injection:
1. Wash and dry hands.
2. Draw required amount of drug up into syringe. Drug, amount and administration must be checked by trained nurse.
3. Carry to bedside. Explain to patient.
4. Expose area (see diagram). Clean skin and hold taut. Insert needle at right angles; withdraw piston slightly to make certain needle is not in deep vein. Push piston home and withdraw needle with swab applied to skin. Massage.
5. Leave patient comfortable.
6. Rinse syringe and needle. Replace in test tube and put aside for resterilisation, unless disposable type has been used.

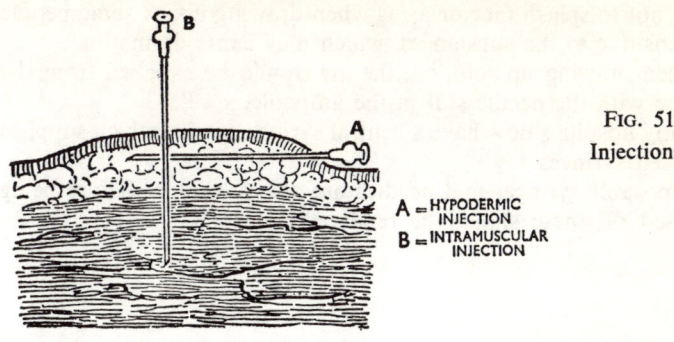

N.B.—Gloves must be worn for giving antibiotics and great care

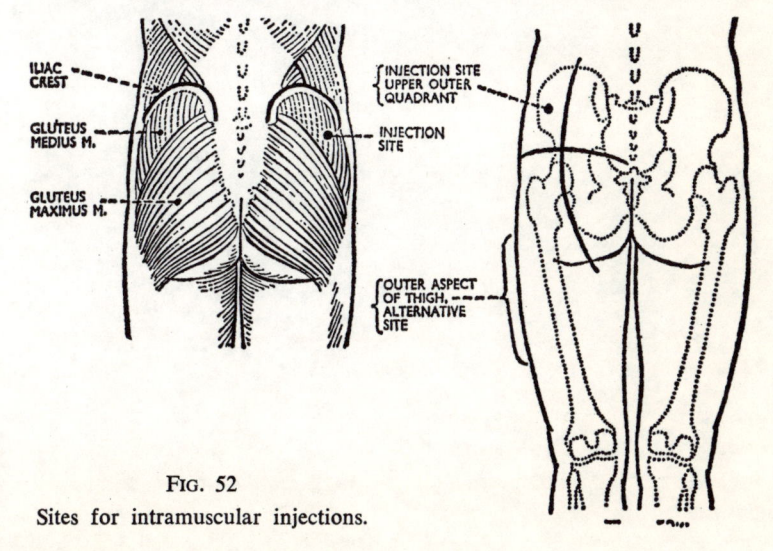

Fig. 52
Sites for intramuscular injections.

taken not to splash face or arms when drawing up, as some people are sensitive to the substances, which may cause dermatitis.

When drawing up solution, the air should be expelled from the syringe with the needle still in the ampoule.

Many hospitals now have a central syringe service which supplies sterilised syringes.

Disposable syringes and needles are also available. Before being disposed of, these should be rendered unusable.

Chapter Nine

INHALATIONS AND OXYGEN

Moist and dry inhalations—Methods of giving oxygen

INHALATIONS

INHALATIONS are used in the treatment of respiratory diseases.

Dry inhalations may be administered, *e.g.* smelling salts. *Moist inhalations* may be given intermittently or continuously.

MOIST INHALATIONS

Nelson's inhaler

Used for intermittent inhalations, 2 to 4 hourly, of warm medicated vapour for inflammation of upper respiratory tract:

1. Common cold.
2. Catarrh.
3. Sinusitis.
4. Laryngitis.
5. Tracheitis.
6. Pharyngitis.

(occasionally in bronchitis and broncho-pneumonia).

Care must be taken that patient is kept in even temperature during course of treatment.

Requirements on a tray:

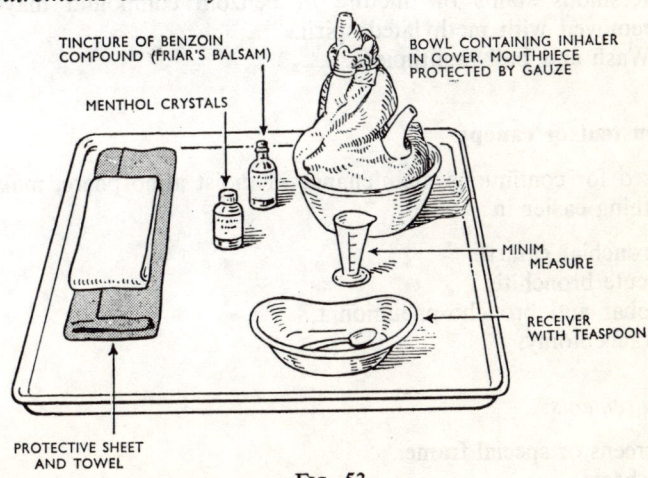

FIG. 53
Tray for moist inhalations.

Preparation of inhaler and medicament:

1. Nearly boiling water, *i.e.* 2 to 3 ounces cold with 16 to 17 ounces boiling water, should be poured in to below level of air inlet (½ to 1 pint according to size of inhaler).
2. Add tincture of benzoin compound, ½ to 1 drachm. Alternative medicaments—pine oil or eucalyptus, ½ to 1 drachm; menthol crystals, 2 or 3.
3. See that mouthpiece is directed away from air inlet.

Method:

1. Explain procedure to patient; close windows if necessary; screen bed.
2. Sit patient well up, support with pillows and place blanket round shoulders.
3. Place bedtable comfortably in front of patient and protect by protective sheet and towel.
4. Place tray containing inhaler on table.
5. Instruct patient not to put fingers over air inlet and to place lips over mouthpiece, to breath in through mouth and out through nose.
6. Patient inhales for 15 to 20 minutes. Paper tissues should be available.
7. A very ill or aged patient, or a child, must never be left.
8. After use, remove apparatus and screens, leaving patient warm and comfortable.
9. Resinous stains of tincture of benzoin compound may be removed with methylated spirit.
10. Wash and boil mouthpiece.

Steam tent or canopy

Used for continuous maintenance of moist atmosphere, making breathing easier in:

1. Bronchial catarrh.
2. Acute bronchitis.
3. Lobar and broncho-pneumonia.
4. Tracheotomy.

Requirements:

1. Screens or special frame.
2. 3 sheets.
3. Room thermometer, placed well away from steam outlet.

INHALATIONS AND OXYGEN

4. Tape and safety pins.
5. Steam kettle standing in tray on floor, spout well away from patient.
6. Jug for refilling kettle.

Kettle refilled and temperature of tent taken every hour; this should not rise above 23·9: C (75° F). Both charted and signed by nurse. If patient is child, watch carefully. Discontinue treatment gradually.

If possible, it is safer if a child is placed in a special cubicle and the kettle kept boiling in a corner of the room, well away from the bed or cot.

More often humidified oxygen is used.

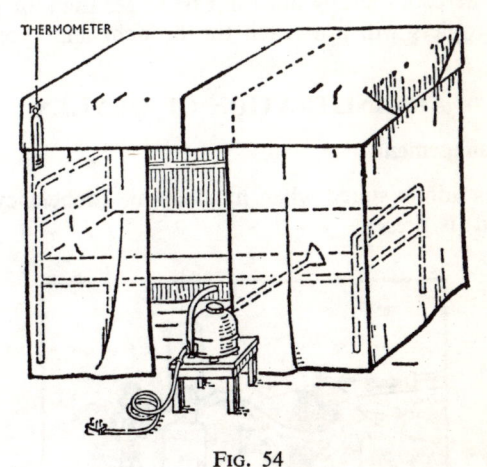

Fig. 54
Steam tent.

DRY INHALATIONS

Ammonia (smelling salts)

Inhaled in cases of fainting; acts by irritating mucous membrane and by reflexly stimulating the respiratory, cardiac and vaso-motor centres, improves circulation.

Amyl nitrate

Used in some forms of angina pectoris. Small capsules are crushed in gauze and held to patient's nose.

Stramonium

Used for relief of asthma; relaxes spasm of bronchial tubes; obtained in cigarette or powder form which is burnt and smoke inhaled.

Aerosol therapy

A detergent spray has been found useful in treating bronchiolitis in children.

The solution is known as Alevaire and is used with an oxygen vaporiser (see Fig. 55). It reduces surface tension of the mucus making it less viscid and more easily expectorated. The mist particles in aerosol therapy must not be larger than 3μ in diameter, as larger droplets will not reach the bronchi and bronchioles.

ADMINISTRATION OF OXYGEN

General management

Oxygen is administered when hypoxaemia (deficiency of oxygen in the blood) is present.

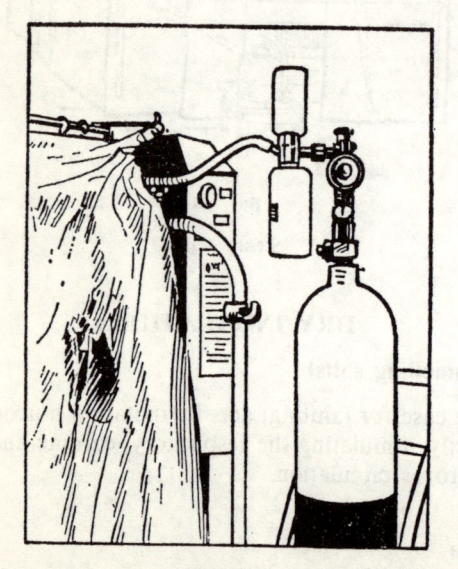

Fig. 55

Oxygen vaporiser.

INHALATIONS AND OXYGEN

Causes of hypoxaemia

1. Cardiac failure.
2. Failure of pulmonary circulation.
3. Pulmonary embolism.
4. Disease of the lung, *e.g.* pneumonia.
5. Chronic lung conditions, *e.g.* emphysema.
6. Severe bleeding and when haemoglobin content of blood is low.
7. Shock and collapse when circulation is depressed.
8. Carbon monoxide poisoning when red cells take up gas instead of oxygen.
9. When absorption of oxygen is reduced at very high altitudes.

Variety of apparatus employed. Ideally, oxygen cylinder should have fine adjustment valve and flowmeter, marked in litres.

Tube and funnel may be used in emergency but is wasteful.

Nasal catheters and nasal tubes on Tudor Edward's spectacle frame or Marriott's headpiece, used with Woulfe's bottle or water flowmeter.

B.L.B. (Boothby, Lovelace and Bulbulian) masks. Plastic masks made by British Oxygen Company or Venturi mask.

Oxygen tents.

Administration of nasal oxygen

Requirements on a tray:

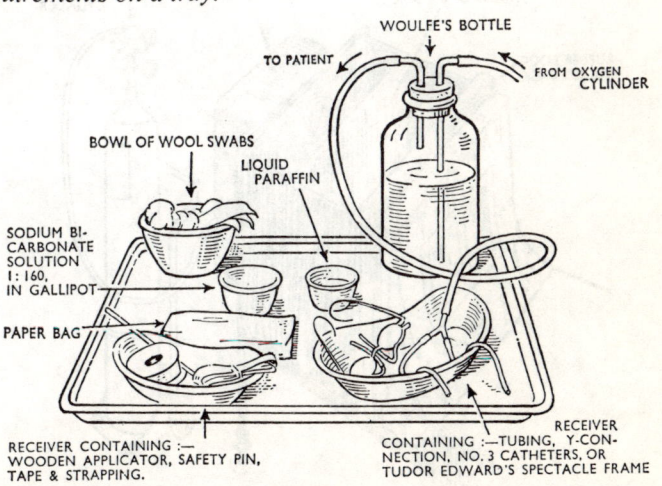

FIG. 56
Tray for administration of nasal oxygen.

Method:

1. If possible explain procedure to patient. Screen bed.
2. Clean nostrils *gently* with a screw of wool on wooden applicator.
3. Regulate flow of oxygen.
4. Lubricate ends of catheter or nasal tubes and gently insert well back into nostrils, passing along floor of nose.
5. Strap catheters to cheeks with small pieces of strapping.
6. Fix tubing to pillow with safety pin and tie excess tubing to head of bed with tape.
7. Leaving patient comfortable, clear away tray and screens.

N.B.—Allow no naked flame or spark in the vicinity when oxygen is being used. Allow no oil or grease to come into contact with pressure gauge fitting. Avoid leaving a gas cylinder close to a radiator.

B.L.B. masks

N.B.—When using nasal pattern mask it is necessary to make sure that patient's nostrils are clear.

The concentration of oxygen depends not only on flow but on use of airports.

Oxygen tents

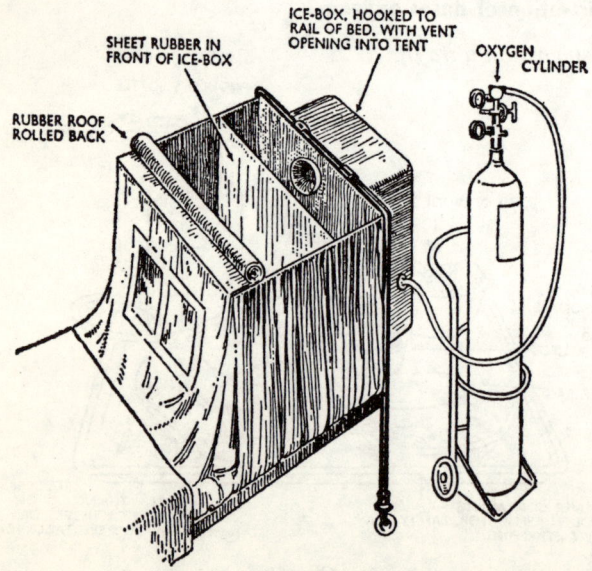

FIG. 57
Oxygen tent, main parts.

Ice is not always necessary in the modern tents.
For cleaning.—1 per cent Dettol in soft water is recommended.

Administration of Carbon Dioxide

Carbon dioxide (CO_2°), 5 per cent or 10 per cent with oxygen is given when ordered to stimulate respiration.

Chapter Ten

PREPARATIONS FOR OPERATION. GENERAL OBSERVATIONS

Preparation of patient for operation—Pre-operative shaving—Care and observation after general anaesthetic—General observation of patient—Care of the unconscious patient

Mental preparation is necessary to overcome natural anxiety. Reassure the patient that all treatment aims at ensuring successful result of the operation. Refer all questions to Sister.

Pre-operative treatment

1. DIET.—*Until day before operation*, usually a liberal diet is given with copious fluids to flush excretory system, *e.g.* Barley water, glucose. *Day before operation*, give a light non-residue diet and fluids. *On operation day*, give last light meal not less than 4 hours before operation and clear fluids up to 2 hours before.

2. CLINICAL EXAMINATION, made by doctor and report given to anaesthetist. *Pre-medication* (drug to aid anaesthetic) is ordered in writing, is given and signed for by a responsible nurse. *Urine* is tested and result charted, abnormalities reported to sister or nurse in charge. Information must be given to anaesthetist.

3. TREATMENT OF THE ALIMENTARY TRACT.—*Mouth*, teeth and throat are attended to previously if possible, to see that there is no oral sepsis. *Stomach* must be empty when anaesthetic is given. *Large intestine* emptied before operation, making sure that bowels are opened day before, if necessary (*a*) by giving full dose of patient's *usual* aperient. (*b*) by giving enema saponis or glycerine suppository on evening before operation.

4. CLEANLINESS OF THE PATIENT.—This applies to hair, skin, nails, umbilicus and perineal area especially.

5. ANY SPECIAL PREPARATION ordered by surgeon is carried out, *e.g.* stomach washout, blood transfusion.

6. LOCAL PREPARATION.—There is a great deal of variation in this procedure, but it may include—shaving, and cleansing of the

skin with soap and water, the use of an antiseptic such as Hibitane. The area may then be covered with a sterile towel or left uncovered.

7. CLOTHING OF PATIENT.—*Requirements:*
Flannel gown, opening at back.
Long woollen stockings, not always used.
Cap or triangular bandage.
2 Theatre blankets.
Stretcher canvas, plastic and draw sheet.

Method:

(*a*) Screen bed and reassure patient.
(*b*) Strip top bedclothes leaving patient covered by blanket. Put patient into gown and stockings if used, remove hair grips, plait hair if long and tie with tape. Put on cap or triangular bandage.
(*c*) Remove dentures, if any, and place in mug of water in locker.
(*d*) Give patient bedpan or urinal. Catheterise if necessary.
(*e*) Place stretcher canvas, plastic and draw sheet in position under patient.
(*f*) Lie patient down and cover with 2 theatre blankets.
(*g*) Give pre-medication and leave patient to rest behind screens.

Collect chart, X-rays, and vomit bowl with cloth and mouth gag, tongue forceps and sponge holder loaded with gauze swab. Accompany patient to theatre. The patient is the responsibility of the nurse and *must not* be left unattended in anaesthetic room.

In anaesthetic room, reassure patient; observe absolute silence during induction. To reassure patient, hold his hands gently, unless otherwise instructed.

Nurse should be able to answer questions about patient, *e.g.* time pre-medication given.

If basal anaesthetic is given in ward, patient must not be left because of danger of obstruction to airway due to relaxation of muscles.

Pre-operative shaving

Requirements on a tray:

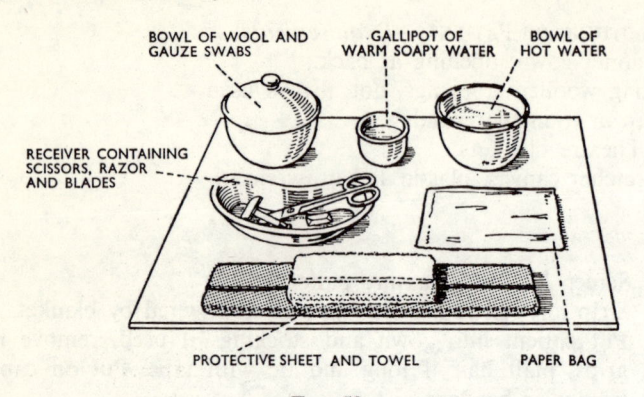

Fig. 58
Tray for pre-operative shaving.

Chest blanket.
The operation site must always be free from hair.

For operations on:

1. Scalp or skull. Whole head is shaved.
2. Ear or mastoid. Area for 3 in. around mastoid process.
3. Eye. Eyebrows only on specific instructions, eyelashes sometimes need to be cut. This needs expert handling and the scissors should be coated with vaseline, to prevent lashes falling into eyes.
4. Breast, shoulder or arm. From below, over shoulder to midline of back and opposite nipple-line in front, also axilla.
5. Upper limb. Whole limb.
6. Abdomen. Lower thorax and whole abdomen including pubes, groins and upper thigh. For hernia operations, whole abdomen below umbilicus, upper thighs, pubes, scrotum or labia and perineum.
7. Vagina, perineum or anus. Complete pubic, perineal and perianal area including inner sides of thighs ('through' shave).
8. Hip. Appropriate side of abdomen, pubes, perineum and whole thigh.
9. Lower limb. Whole limb.

Shaving is carried out by the nurse, for female patients. For male patients either a male nurse, orderly or barber performs the shave. Sparse hair, such as that on limbs is best removed with a dry razor. Longer hair, *e.g.* pubic or axillary, should be cut short with scissors before lathering with soap and shaving with the razor.

The procedure of shaving, particularly a 'through' shave, is embarrassing for patient; therefore great care should be taken to expose as little of patient as possible.

Commence a 'through' shave with patient in the dorsal position, but complete in left lateral position.

SKIN PREPARATION.—After shaving, some surgeons consider that bathing or washing the area with soap and water is sufficient, followed by the use of antiseptics at time of operation; others require that the skin should be prepared with antiseptic in the ward.

In this case a dressing trolley is required and the skin is prepared by thorough cleansing with a detergent, such as Cetrimide or Bradosol, particular attention being paid to the umbilicus and creases such as the groin. The skin is then painted with the desired antiseptic, allowed to dry and covered with a sterile cloth which is bandaged in position.

N.B. If iodine is used, it must be allowed to dry thoroughly. Also it is wise to do a small iodine sensitivity test on inner side of thigh.

Post-operative care

Post-operation bed made as soon as patient has left ward. (See Chapter III, Bedmaking.)

Sufficient helpers must be available to lift patient from trolley to bed. If on stretcher, canvas left in position until patient has recovered from anaesthetic. Patient is placed flat on back with head turned to one side or on right side with pillow supporting back. Bed elevator placed in position if necessary.

Patient must not be left until completely recovered from anaesthetic. Airway not removed until cough reflex returns.

OBSERVATIONS:

1. Pulse rate and quality ($\frac{1}{4}$ or $\frac{1}{2}$ hourly chart kept as ordered).
2. Respiration rate and character.
3. Blood pressure.
4. Colour.
5. Patient's movements; if restless, restrain gently; prevent injury.
6. Mouth and throat must be kept clear of mucus and vomit.
7. See that any drainage tube is kept free and working.
8. Note the condition of dressing.

After recovery from anaesthetic and shock, patient is washed and put into own bed-wear. Mouthwash given and patient placed into comfortable position as directed.

Sips of water may be given unless contra-indicated.

Note made of passage of urine, measured.

Watch dressing, particularly if any drainage.

Pain and restlessness reported and treated by the administration of drugs as ordered.

Later, patient is encouraged to move legs and breathe deeply. Exercises, general and breathing may be ordered and given. Time in bed depends on condition of patient and wishes of surgeon.

If spinal anaesthetic has been given and blood pressure lowered, bed may be elevated for several hours after administration and then gradually sit patient up, adding one pillow at a time, to avoid collapse. Watch returning movement in lower extremities.

Post-anaesthetic recovery rooms are now often used.

GENERAL OBSERVATION TO BE MADE OF PATIENTS

The best observations are the simple ones which are recorded with accuracy. They are made by what the nurse may see, hear, feel and smell.

Things to notice:

1. General attitude.
2. Posture and gait.
3. Mental condition, whether cheerful or depressed.
4. Appearance of comfort or pain.
5. Warm or cold.
6. Trembling or shivering.
7. Clean or dirty.
8. Fat or thin.
9. Colour of skin.
10. Crying, groaning or sighing.
11. Character of breathing.
12. Odour from mouth, body or clothing.
13. Position in bed.
14. Presence of rashes, scars or deformity.
15. Sleep.
16. Any special complaints by patient.

CARE OF THE UNCONSCIOUS PATIENT

The care of the unconscious patient, his very life in fact, depends entirely on the nurse. Today, increasing road accidents, with severe injuries, have meant an increase in unconscious patients on the wards. (First care will be one of transport, *e.g.* from casualty to the ward, or operating theatre to the ward). The nurse is responsible for the safety of the patient during transfer, and must always ensure a *clear airway*, make sure that the patient's limbs are not injured in transit, ensure warmth in draughty corridors, also make sure if possible that she has all the patient's belongings.

On arrival at the ward the patient must be carefully lifted from the trolley to the bed (enough help being obtained to ensure this, jolting may increase shock) and placed in a suitable position (usually semiprone) but may be flat on the back with the head to one side, sometimes foot of bed is elevated to allow secretions to leave the mouth and not block the airway.

Continuous observance should be made, and the patient must not be left even for a moment, care should be taken to prevent further injury, *e.g.* if the patient's eyes are open make sure the bedclothes do not rub against them, or a hair get into them (brush hair well back). The most important observation is to ensure that the airway is maintained, it must be kept clear and any mucus, blood or vomit cleared with sponge holding forceps dressed with gauze swabs, or the use of a suction apparatus. Cyanosis and any unusual sound (rattling) in the unconscious patient means that obstruction is present. Respiration, pulse and blood pressure must be carefully recorded at intervals ordered by the doctor.

Any patient who is unconscious will need special care of their limbs to avoid undue stretching which may cause foot drop and permanent damage to the muscles. If the limbs are placed in a position of relaxation, this will not occur, *i.e.* roll in the hand, arms abducted, legs in correct position. Footboards and sandbags can help in keeping the limbs in position.

The physiotherapist helps to prevent respiratory complications and muscle damage, but the nurse is the person who deals mainly with the patient, so she must take as many preventive measures as possible.

If the state of unconsciousness is prolonged (head injury) then other procedures will be needed. Fluids must be given (by some other route than the mouth, often intravenously). Dehydration must not be allowed to occur, and fluids will be needed quickly if the patient perspires profusely or has pyrexia.

It is essential to change his position frequently, to prevent pressure sores, and special care of the bladder and bowels will be necessary.

The patient may be restless, in which case sedatives will be ordered by the doctor, and cot sides may be used.

WRITING REPORTS

At top:

Number of empty beds.
Names of admissions and discharges and where to.

GENERAL REPORTS.—*Day:*

(*a*) *New patients:* age, religion, diagnosis, emergency or 'written for' case, name of physician or surgeon in charge, general condition and treatment carried out or to be done.

(*b*) *Ill patients:* general condition, temperature, pulse and respiration, drugs, special treatment, X-rays or other investigations done or to be done, diet, vomits, urine and bowels open; whether relatives have enquired.

(*c*) *Post-operation.*—Pre-operative drugs given and time; time patient went to theatre; duration of operation and condition of patient during it; nature of operation; post-operative condition of patient, immediate and later; drugs given with time of giving; whether passed urine, vomiting, temperature, pulse and respiration, dressing, diet, position, special treatment, enquiry by relatives.

Night.—Sleep, general condition, treatment given, drugs given, temperature, pulse and respiration, emergencies.

The Kardex system is now being widely used for reports.

General nursing care

Includes cleanliness of body, hands and feet, head and hair, mouth and teeth. Diet and serving of meals. Giving bedpans and urinals and observation of excreta. Making beds and comfort of patient. General interest in patient and occupation given to ensure patient does not become bored.

Attitude towards patient admitted for few hours, *e.g.* for special test or treatment, one of welcome and reassurance.

Chapter Eleven

PREPARATION OF PATIENT FOR VARIOUS EXAMINATIONS

Physical—X-ray—Radium therapy—Endoscopy—Dilatation and curettage

FOR PHYSICAL EXAMINATION

For all examinations.—Explain procedure to patient, screen bed and shut windows if necessary.

Eye

Room should be darkened if possible; if not, lower blinds on either side of bed. Light above and opposite surgeon. It may be necessary to steady patient's head. Ophthalmoscope should be available.

Ear

Requirements on a tray:

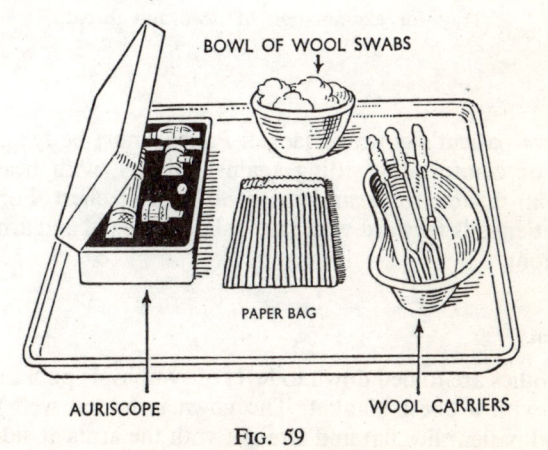

FIG. 59
Tray for examination of the ear.

Affected ear should be turned towards the doctor. Steady head.

Nose and throat

Patient should face the doctor. Light either by torch or head mirror and place lamp behind and above patient's shoulder.

N.B.—If possible patients are taken to an Ear, Nose and Throat Clinic. Patient sits on chair facing the surgeon. There is a light behind and above the patient's right shoulder. Nurse stands behind patient and steadies head if necessary.

Requirements on a tray:

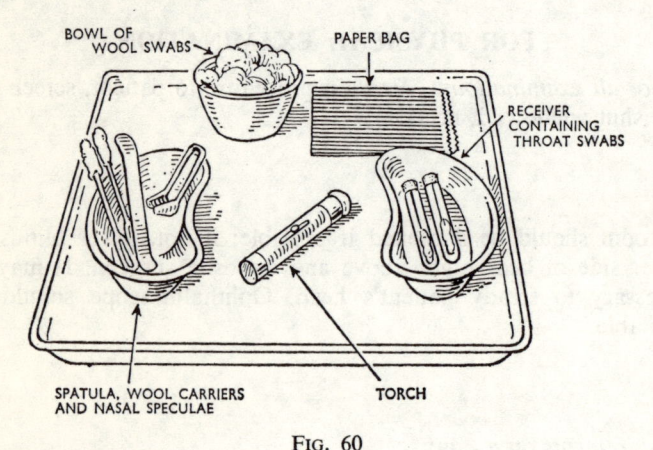

FIG. 60
Tray for examination of nose and throat.

Chest

Remove patient's gown or jacket. Patient must be lying flat and straight or comfortably sitting against pillows, with head turned away from doctor, for examination of front of chest. For back of chest, patient sits forward with knees slightly flexed and arms folded across front.

Abdomen

Bedclothes are folded down to level of symphysis pubis, and chest covered with a chest blanket. The gown is folded well up on to chest and patient lies flat and straight with the arms at sides.

Rectum

Requirements on a tray:

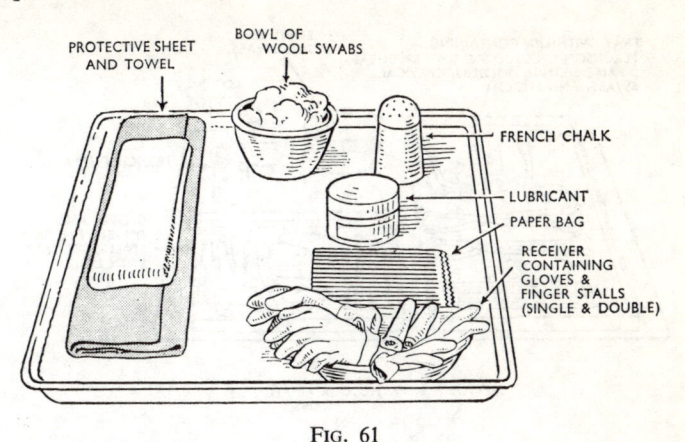

FIG. 61
Tray for rectal examination.

Turn down bedclothes to level of symphysis pubis; see that chest is covered by a blanket. Patient should lie in left lateral position with buttocks to edge of bed. Protective sheet and towel are placed under buttocks.

Vagina

Requirements on a trolley:

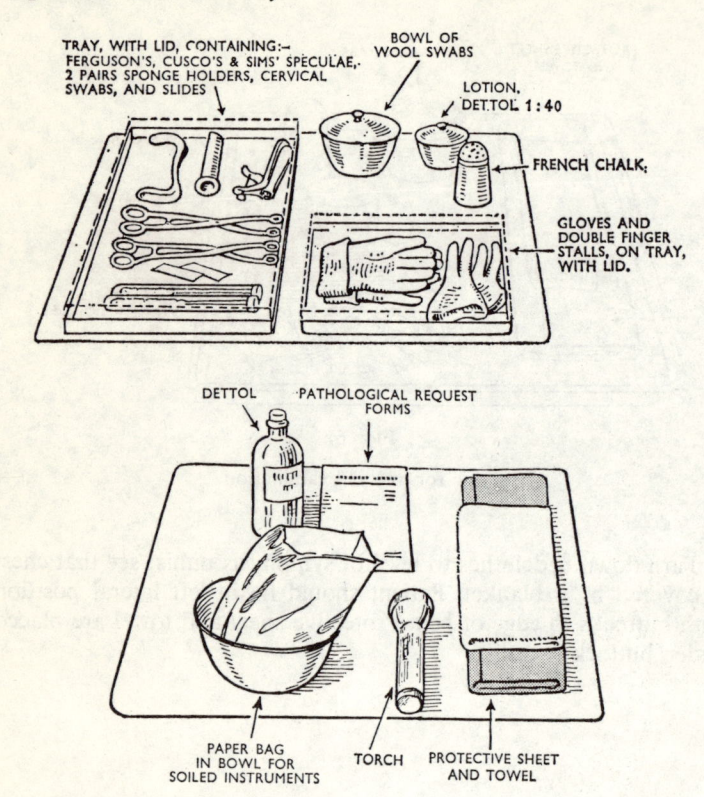

FIG. 62

Trolley for examination of vagina.

Patient is given bedpan. Bedclothes are turned down to the knees and the chest covered by a blanket. Patient's nightdress is turned well up to chest. Protective sheet and towel are placed under buttocks.

POSITIONS.—Dorsal, Sim's, left lateral, knee-chest.

Nervous system

Requirements on a tray:

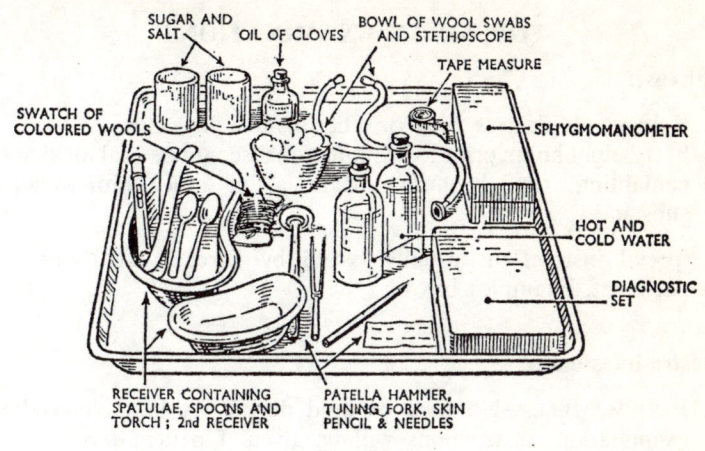

FIG. 63

Tray for examination of nervous system.

Patient is examined up and in bed.

General physical examination

Light must be good; room warm; patient comfortable.

INSPECTION PROVIDES INFORMATION ABOUT:

1. General condition of patient's body.
2. State of nutrition.
3. Any deformities, rashes, injuries, irregularities or other marks.
4. Colour and character of skin.
5. State of eyes, *e.g.* bloodshot, jaundiced.
6. Presence of pallor or cyanosis.
7. Any distressing symptoms, *e.g.* dyspnoea, restlessness, twitchings.

INSPECTION MAY INCLUDE:

Palpation (Touch).—Alterations and variations in development found, *e.g.* shape of chest. Size and character of tumours.
Percussion (Tapping).—Alteration in sound over organs, *e.g.* whether lungs sound resonant (air present) or dull (fluid present).
Auscultation (Listening).—Sounds of heart and lungs. When

stethoscope being used there should be no friction or rub between clothing.

FOR X-RAY EXAMINATIONS

All cases
1. Remove all plasters, pins, or other opaque dressings.
2. Forty-eight hours prior to examination discontinue oral medicines containing iron, bismuth, magnesia, or other radio-opaque substance.

Special instructions usually issued by Director of Radiology Department. Examples below:

Gastro-intestinal
1. BARIUM MEAL.—No food or fluid during six hours preceding examination. Instructions will be given if patient has to continue fasting prior to further examination.
2. BARIUM ENEMA.—A high colonic washout to be given not less than four hours before examination, or 1 Dulcolax tablet, two consecutive evenings before and 1 Dulcolax suppository on morning of X-ray examination.

Excretion urography
1. No fluid at all during six hours preceding examination.
2. No heavy meals during six hours preceding examination: light meals may be given, but should not include any food containing a large proportion of water, *e.g.* porridge, jelly, junket, etc.
3. When possible, patients confined to bed should be given high colonic washout on second evening before examination, and an aperient, on night before examination.

Cholecystography
1. An ordinary meal to be given at 6 p.m. on day preceding examination.
2. At 7 p.m. the opaque medium should be given in accordance with directions on bottle.
3. After that no further fluid or food until after examination.
4. After first examination one egg beaten up in glass of warm milk to be given, unless otherwise arranged by X-ray Department.

Aortography and cardiac catheterisation

Preferably undertaken on the conscious patient, but babies and young children may require a general anaesthetic.

All patients require sedation, this may be carried out by the use of various drugs, *e.g.* Omnopon and scopolomine for young children, dose according to age. A barbiturate such as Sodium amytal for older children and adults, again, dosage according to age.

If the femoral artery is used it may be necessary to shave the patient.

FOR RADIUM THERAPY

Radium is a radio-active substance made up of atoms and particles having a high velocity. It disintegrates slowly and presents a constant source of radio-activity. *Rays emitted are:* alpha, beta and gamma. Gamma have the greatest powers of penetration in tissues and are employed for therapeutic purposes. They are similar to X-rays.

Radon is gas given off. It is collected in tubes or seeds. As it disintegrates in a few days, it is useful for out-patients.

Effect of radium on tissues

This was first shown on workers carrying radium in trouser pockets. Inflammation and destruction of tissues of thigh resulted.

In therapeutic practice some tumours are found to be more sensitive than others. Cells are more vulnerable when rapidly dividing, rapidly growing tumours are, therefore, more susceptible. Cells of sex glands divide more rapidly than any others in the body. Blood forming organs are very susceptible to radium. Susceptibility of tissue also depends on presence of connective tissue and blood supply.

Cancer cells are killed by radium. The growth of connective tissue is stimulated, resulting in formation of fibrous tissue which contracts and by pressure and strangulation help to destroy cancer cells.

The *radiologist* is concerned with the provision of the correct dose of radium for each patient. Alpha and beta rays which are more destructive to healthy tissue than cancerous must be cut out and the therapy of the diseased area limited to gamma rays.

The *nurse* working in the Radiotherapy Department is concerned with the knowledge that the skin is more sensitive to radium than deeper structures and her duty lies in the carrying out of instructions provided about protection of the skin.

Application of radium

1. Careful calculation and regulation for each patient.
2. Alpha rays very irritating to tissues; do not travel far; stopped by slight protection, *e.g.* piece of paper.
3. Beta rays sometimes used in treatment of warts and of tumours; layer of platinum stops their penetration.
4. Gamma rays have selective action on tumour cells; will pass through several inches of lead; penetrate fairly deeply into tissues.
5. Applied on specially prepared applicators, in platinum or gold screens. Radon applied in small tubes of glass, called seeds.

Radium reaction, which may occur

1. Redness, irritation and pain.
2. Tingling of skin, few days after application.
3. Inflammation proceeds, maximum in two weeks.
4. Skin very red and covered with exudate. Blisters and peels.

Treatment.—Bland applications, *e.g.* Lanoline may be used or a simple dusting powder.

Symptoms of prolonged radiation

1. Headache and giddiness.
2. Loss of appetite.
3. Nausea and vomiting.
4. Diarrhoea.
5. Malaise.
6. Anaemia.
7. Toxaemia.

Diet should be very nutritious.

General indications during treatment

1. Confine to an area, if possible in a cubicle.
2. Have special label on bed or door of cubicle.
3. See that container is at hand for loose needles.
4. See that application is maintained in position.
5. Attend particularly to patient's comfort.
6. Warn patient not to touch area.
7. Inspect bedpans, if treatment in lower region.
8. Use no metallic substances; makes skin more sensitive.

Protection of nursing staff

1. All staff wear special exposure film badges.
2. Should have regular blood counts to eliminate possibility of anaemia.
3. Fresh air and good food essential.
4. Handle radium as little as possible.
5. Stay at bedside for as short a time as possible.

RADIOACTIVE ISOTOPES

Isotope.—A variation of an element, with identical chemical property but a different atomic weight.

Most elements have at least two isotopes.

Radioactive isotopes are isotopes of certain elements produced artificially by bombardment of the nuclei of the atoms in an atomic pile. These are used medically in certain conditions:

1. *Radioactive iodine*, used in the treatment of carcinoma of the thyroid. Given by mouth and absorbed into the bloodstream through the alimentary tract. Deposited in the thyroid gland from the bloodstream it acts as a source of localised radiation. It is usually given in sufficient doses to obliterate all active thyroid tissue and also to be taken up by any secondary deposits of malignant cells.
2. *Radioactive phosphorus*, used in the treatment of polycythemia (excessive number of red blood cells). Given by mouth or intravenous injection.
3. *Radioactive cobalt*, used in the treatment of carcinoma instead of 'bomb' or beam unit. Has long 'life' compared with other radioactive isotopes, losing half its strength in rather more than five years.
4. *Radioactive gold*, used in the treatment of malignant diseases which cause large peritoneal or pleural effusions, to save the patient from considerable discomfort by reducing the effusion. It may also be introduced into the peritoneal cavity if there is a possibility of 'overspill' of malignant cells, *e.g.* from an ovarian cyst.

RADIOACTIVE TRACERS.—The Geiger counter is a delicate instrument used to detect minute quantities of radioactive substance.

E.g.—Radioactive iodine can be used to assess activity of thyroid gland, a small dose being given by mouth, the Geiger counter is then put in position over the thyroid gland, this will record the arrival of the radioactive isotopes in the gland tissue.

If there is no active thyroid tissue, no iodine will be taken up.

If there is enlargement or increased activity of the gland then the rate of absorption of iodine will be greater than normal.

PRECAUTIONS.—Similar precautions to those in use for the handling of radium and X-rays are necessary. In addition it is necessary to work behind screens, wear protective clothing including rubber gloves, as there is danger of contamination with radioactive particles. No eating, drinking or smoking should be allowed during the use of these substances.

Patients receiving doses of radioactive isotopes excrete some of the material in their urine, therefore nursing staff dealing with bedpans and urinals should wear protective clothing and rubber gloves. The radioactive urine must be stored in large bottles or tanks in a lead-lined cupboard for a suitable length of time, *i.e.* until the isotopes become inactive. After which it can be disposed of in the usual way.

The length of time taken by radioactive isotopes to decay differs with the elements concerned.

FOR ENDOSCOPY

Preparation of equipment for endoscopies is dealt with under Operating Theatre Technique.

Meaning of, and preparation of patient for:

1. SIGMOIDOSCOPY.—(*a*) Examination of sigmoid colon and rectum, using a long tubular speculum with a light at the far end, called a sigmoidoscope. Folds of mucous membrane fall against the end of the instrument so air inflation is used during introduction to prevent obstruction of view.

    (*b*) Some surgeons require minimum amount of preparation of patient, *i.e.* enema given the previous evening; others prefer rectal washout to be carried out until fluid returns clear.

2. CYSTOSCOPY.—(*a*) Examination of urinary bladder with a cystoscope which is a simple, very narrow telescope into which is built a light and prism to enable field of vision to cover a wide area.

    (*b*) Apart from personal hygiene of the external genital organs there is usually no other preparation. Some surgeons prefer patient to be shaved.

3. OESOPHAGOSCOPY AND GASTROSCOPY.—(*a*) Examination of oesophagus with an oesophagoscope, which is similar in construction to a sigmoidoscope, and examination of the inside

of the stomach with a gastroscope which has a flexible end. Air inflation is used for these procedures.

(b) *For oesophagoscopy* patient is prepared for a general anaesthetic. Local preparation consists of gently irrigating oesophagus through a Ryle's tube, rubber catheter or oesophageal tube.

A gastroscopy is usually carried out under premedication such as morphine and atropine (latter being most important to abolish flow of saliva), and a local anaesthetic, *e.g.* amethocaine, 2 ml being used and dropped on to patient's lips from a hypodermic syringe, patient being instructed to move it around mouth and then swallow. In two minutes whole mouth and oesophagus is anaesthetised. It may be necessary for patient to have a stomach washout before premedication, as stomach must be empty.

4. LARYNGOSCOPY AND BRONCHOSCOPY.—(*a*) Examination of the larynx or bronchi with a laryngoscope or bronchoscope which is similar to an oesophagoscope.

(b) No preparation of the patient is necessary except by premedication, this being followed by local anaesthesia.

Sometimes the procedure is carried out under general anaesthesia, when patient must be prepared accordingly.

5. THORACOSCOPY AND PERITONEOSCOPY.—(*a*) Examinations of inside of thorax and peritoneal cavity respectively, using an instrument similar to a cystoscope and passing it through a small incision in chest or abdominal wall.

(b) Apart from premedication there is no preparation of patient as procedure is carried out under local anaesthetic.

FOR DILATION AND CURETTAGE

Therapeutic and diagnostic.

Under general anaesthesia the cervix of the uterus is dilated with special metal bougies and the uterine cavity scraped with a curette. Pieces of the lining membrane may be sent for microscopic examination.

Preparation of the patient includes:

1. Enema saponis, or glycerine suppository.
2. 'Through' shave and cleansing of vulva and perineum.
3. Catheterisation.
4. Sometimes packing of vagina with ribbon gauze and antiseptic.

Instruments required:

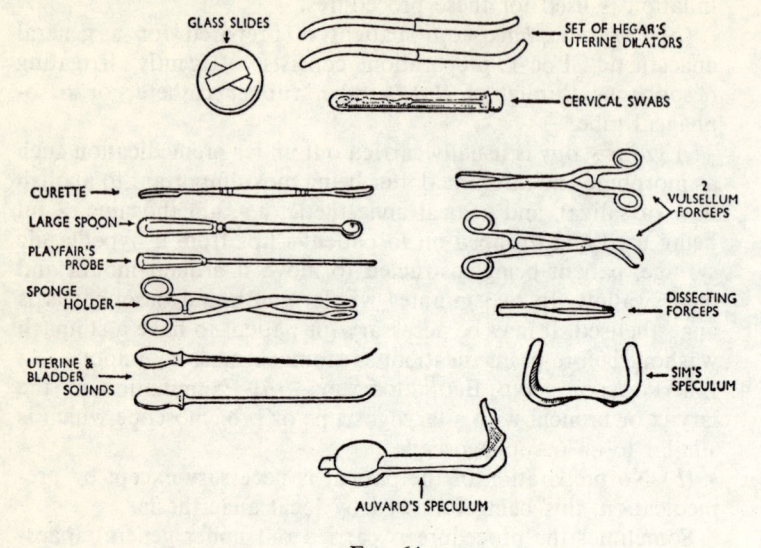

Fig. 64

Instruments of dilatation and curettage.

Chapter Twelve

LOCAL APPLICATIONS. BATHS

*Cold—Hot—Counter-irritants—Miscellaneous—
Medicated baths—Sponging*

Before any procedure, explain to patient and screen bed in each case.

COLD

Applications of cold contract superficial blood vessels and check inflammation in early stages, by inhibiting activity of bacteria and preventing their multiplication. By lessening supply of blood to part swelling is reduced or prevented. Cold also reduces temperature and assists in controlling haemorrhage. It numbs nerve endings and so relieves pain.

Cold compress

Requirements on a tray:

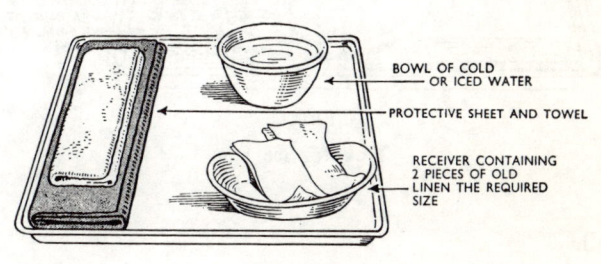

FIG. 65
Tray for cold compress.

Method:
1. Expose area and place protective sheet and towel.
2. Place old linen in iced water, lightly wring one piece out, and place over affected area.
3. Leave second piece of old linen in readiness for changing. Pieces are changed frequently, to keep them cold and moist over the prescribed length of time.
4. When applications are finished, dry part and leave patient comfortable.
5. Clear away tray and screens.

Evaporating compress

This is carried out in same way as above, but methylated spirit or eau de cologne is added to water, equal parts being used, to give more rapidly evaporating mixture and consequently quicker chilling effect.

Various other evaporating lotions may be used, *e.g.* lead and opium.

Ice bag

Requirements on a tray:

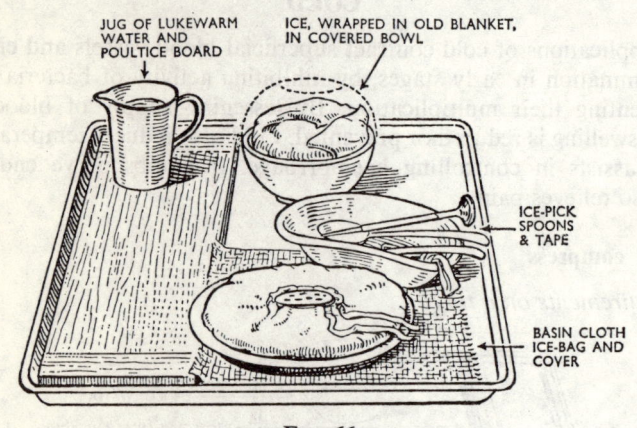

FIG. 66
Tray for ice bag.

Cradle.

Method:

1. Crack ice by pressure with ice pick or pin between two pieces of old blanket on poultice board.
2. Place in bowl of water to round edges.
3. Fill icebag half full.
4. Expel air and screw in cap.
5. Dry outside of bag which may have become wet from condensation of water vapour in atmosphere. Put into cover.
6. Carry to bedside on tray, with cradle and tape.
7. Suspend from cradle over part, so that ice bag is resting lightly on skin.

8. Refill when ice has melted. Discontinue if part becomes discoloured as gangrene and frostbite may occur.

Icebag must be emptied and dried after use. Powder inside with French chalk and inflate slightly. Store flat.

HOT

Applications of heat dilate the superficial blood vessels so increasing the supply of blood to the part (hyperaemia). It also increases number and activity of leucocytes, favouring suppuration and removal of waste products. Heat causes relaxation of muscles; is commonly employed to relieve pain and congestion.

Simple applications of heat may be carried out by use of hot water bottles, hot baths, bathing with hot water, electric pads and cradles. Great care must be taken against burning.

Surgical fomentation

Sterile. Applied to broken skin surface.

Requirements as for surgical dressing with additions on a tray:

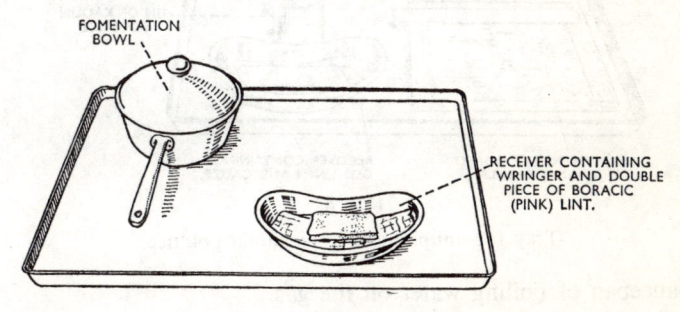

FIG. 67
Tray for surgical fomentation.

Method:

1. Boil fomentation for 5 minutes to render sterile. Use special saucepan or fomentation bowl.
2. Expose wound and clean in usual way.
3. Assistant fetches fomentation in bowl on tray, wrings out, and unfolds wringer.

4. Dresser picks up fomentation with dressing forceps and shakes; applies it to wound, covering with white wool (sterile). Fixes it in position with bandage.
5. Patient is made comfortable and equipment cleared away.

A surgical fomentation requires changing ½ to 2 hourly as ordered.

Poultice (cataplasm)

Substance is mixed to soft consistency with boiling water and spread on cloth. Substances used include, bread or starch.

Antiphlogistine or kaolin, a ready prepared poultice, is more commonly used nowadays.

ANTIPHLOGISTINE OR KAOLIN.—A preparation of china clay containing volatile oils including methylsalicylate.

Requirements on a tray:

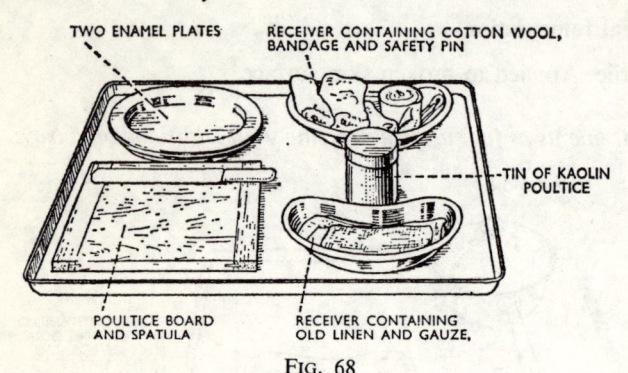

FIG. 68
Tray for antiphlogistine or kaolin poultice.

Saucepan of boiling water on the gas.

Method:

1. Spread kaolin on old linen and cover with gauze.
2. Place between two enamel plates, and stand on top of saucepan of boiling water to heat.
3. Prepare area; fetch poultice and before applying, test on back of hand.
4. Cover with cotton wool and bandage.
5. Make patient comfortable. Clear equipment.

This application does not require such frequent changing as other poultices because of its heat-retaining properties—6 to 8 hourly is usually sufficient. May be reheated once.

STARCH POULTICE.—Used to remove dried crusts in skin conditions, *e.g.* impetigo.

Requirements on a tray:

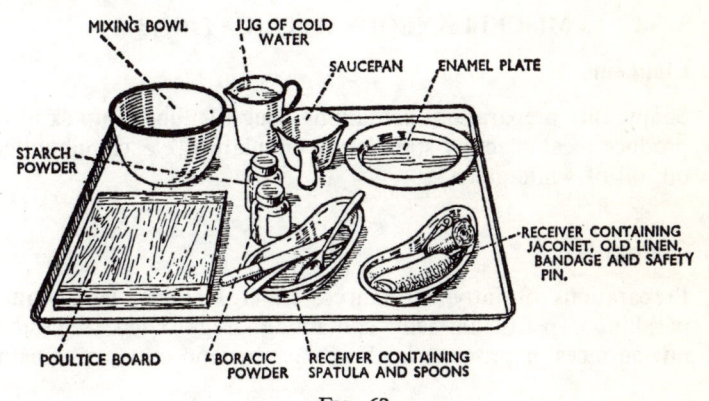

FIG. 69
Tray for starch poultice.

Supply of boiling water.

Method:

1. Measure out starch powder into mixing bowl and add boracic powder (1½ tablespoonfuls of starch, 1 drachm of boracic powder, to approximately 10 oz of water).
2. Mix to smooth paste with little cold water.
3. Add boiling water, stirring all the time, until starch clears.
4. Boil for two minutes, if necessary to make thicker.
5. Allow to cool slightly.
6. Spread about ¾ inch thick on to old linen, place on enamel plate and carry to bedside on tray.
7. Apply poultice to area when nearly cold, cover with jaconet and bandage in position.
8. Leave poultice in position for 6 to 12 hours, after which take off gently; using olive oil, wool swabs and dissecting forceps, carefully remove remaining scabs.
9. Apply dressing as ordered.

COUNTER-IRRITANTS

These are substances which produce superficial irritation or inflammation with the object of relieving pain or congestion of deeper tissues. They are classified according to the effects they produce, rubefacients, causing reddening of the skin, *e.g.* camphor; vesicants, producing blistering of the skin, *e.g.* cantharides.

MISCELLANEOUS APPLICATIONS

1. Liniments

Soapy, oily preparations containing drugs. Rubbed into skin, to produce local effect by stimulating circulation, *e.g.* camphorated oil, oil of wintergreen.

2. Ointments

Preparations of fatty substances, either lanoline, lard, liquid paraffin or petroleum jelly containing drugs. Used to protect raw surfaces or promote healing, *e.g.* zinc and castor oil cream.

3. Scott's dressing

An application of mercury used for treatment of inflammation of joints (synovitis). Strips of lint covered with ointment applied over area; these in turn covered by strips of adhesive plaster; whole application then covered by firm bandage.

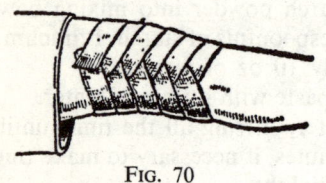

FIG. 70

Scott's dressing applied to knee joint.

4. Unna's Paste

A mixture of gelatine, glycerine and zinc powder. Applied as dressing and support for varicose ulcers.
Prepared bandages now available, *e.g.* Viscopaste.

N.B.—3 and 4 rarely used nowadays.

BATHS

Baths are ordered for the following reasons:

1. To cleanse.
2. To stimulate the action of the skin.
3. To act as a sedative.
4. To reduce temperature.
5. To treat special conditions, *e.g.* skin conditions, stiffness, burns, resuscitating new-born baby, convulsions, mental disorders.

Temperatures of baths

      Cold   —10° to 21·1° C (50° to 70° F).
      Tepid —21·1° to 32·2° C (70° to 90° F).
      Warm —32·2° to 37·8° C (90° to 100° F).
      Hot   —37·8° to 43·3° C (100° to 110° F).
      Vapour—40·6° to 48·9° C (105° to 120° F).
      Hot air—46·1° to 71·1° C (115° to 160° F).

Varieties of baths

VAPOUR BATH.

TURKISH BATH.

MEDICATED BATHS.

1. *Emollient.*—Used in cases of skin irritation.
 Substances used: powdered borax, ½ lb to 30 gallons. Sodium bicarbonate, 1 lb to 30 gallons.
2. *Antiseptic.*—Used for relief of parasitic skin conditions.
 Substance used: sulphur 2 to 3 oz to 30 gallons.

STIMULATING BATHS.—Used to increase the circulation in the subcutaneous tissues, believed to have a tonic effect on general system.
Types used: Cold bath; sea water, 7 lb sea salt to bath; mustard, 1 lb to bath.

AERATED BATH.—Air under pressure is passed into water. Bubbles of air rising to the surface cause movement. Stimulates skin; causes heart to beat faster and increase tone of cardiac muscle. Body functions generally improved; gives sense of well-being.

FOAM BATH.—In medicine, foam-producing herb used, 1 to 2 oz plus aerating apparatus. Gas, CO_2 or oxygen, or air under pressure passed through; increases activity of skin.

SPONGING

Either tepid water (tepid sponging) between 23·9° and 26·7° C (75° and 80° F), or cold water (cold sponging) below 21·1° C (70° F), may be used for the reduction of temperature in cases of hyperpyrexia.

This is not the same as hypothermia.

Requirements on a trolley:

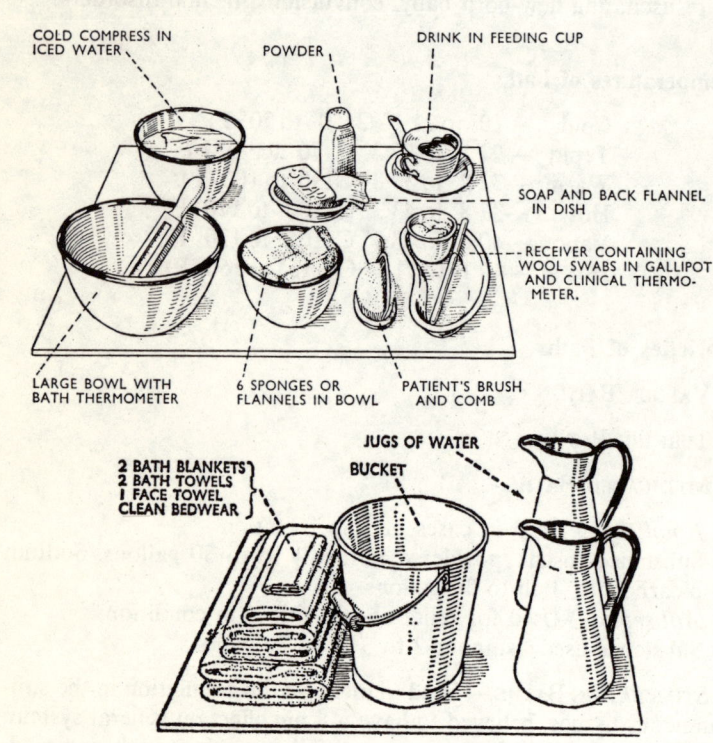

FIG. 71
Trolley for sponging.

Method:

Patient stripped between bath blankets.
Face sponged and dried.
Sponges then placed in axillae and groins (changed frequently), nurse using other two alternately. Sponge upper extremities first with wet sponge and long slow strokes leaving droplets of water on

skin. Allow skin to dry. Front of body treated next then lower extremities. Lastly patient turned and back sponged after which pressure areas may be treated. Whenever possible during treatment cold compress should be kept on the patient's forehead. Temperature taken ten minutes after sponging, fall of 1 to 2° C considered satisfactory. General condition carefully observed.

Electric fans may be used to cool patient by creating air circulation.

Chapter Thirteen

EXTENSIONS. PLASTER OF PARIS. SPLINTS

EXTENSIONS

Extension of a part is achieved by traction, *i.e.* pulling by means of weights attached to the part.

Indications for traction

1. To overcome muscle spasm, *e.g.* damage to central nervous system.
2. To overcome and prevent over-riding of fragments of bone, *e.g.* fracture.
3. To separate joint surfaces and so limit spread of disease, *e.g.* tuberculosis of knee joint.

Counter-traction must always be provided or patient will merely slip down in bed and 'pull' or traction will be lost.

It may be provided by

1. Elevating foot of bed on bed elevator, so using patient's own weight as counter-traction, *e.g.* Byrant's apparatus.
2. Attaching cord and weight to top of Thomas' splint or well-padded groin strap round good leg to top of bed.

Types of traction

1. Balanced or sliding, when weights and pulleys are used.
2. Fixed, when webbing straps or bandages attached to limb are tied to end of splint, as in first-aid.

Traction may be applied in two ways: (1) by skin; (2) by skeleton.

Skin traction is applied by means of strapping, elastoplast or Ventfoam and part must be shaved.

Skeletal traction is obtained by inserting a pin or wire through a bone in an aseptic manner.

POINTS TO NOTE IN NURSING PATIENTS WITH TRACTION

1. Traction must *never* be released whatever the purpose.
2. Pressure sores must be avoided by conscientious routine care of danger areas.

EXTENSIONS. PLASTER OF PARIS. SPLINTS

3. If splints incorporating leather are used treat leather with saddle soap at least once daily to keep supple.
4. Extensions must be inspected at least twice a day to ensure good position, proper pull, and that moisture is not collecting.
5. Weights must hang clear and not rest against anything.
6. Any exposed part must be kept warm, protected from weight of the bedclothes; if a leg, the ankle must be dorsi- and plantar-flexed at least three times daily.
7. A lifting pulley and air-ring may be allowed.

Skeletal traction is applied through the femoral condyles, femoral shaft, upper or lower end of tibia or in the upper limb, through the olecranon process.

A general anaesthetic will be required; for necessary equipment see Anaesthetics, Chapter XXII.

Extension requirements on a trolley:

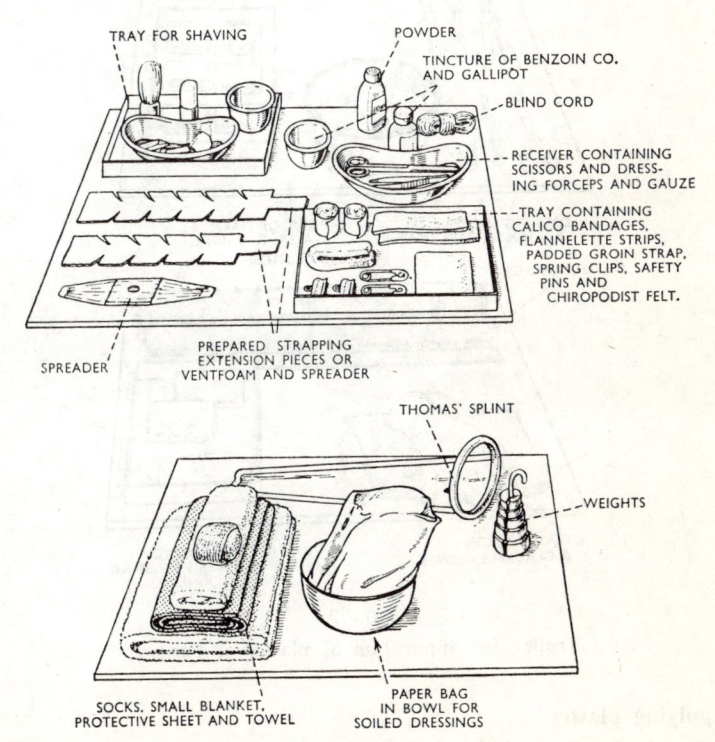

Fig. 72
Trolley for extension requirements.

Fracture boards on bed. Bed elevator.
Extension packs are now available for both adults and children.

PLASTER OF PARIS

A white powder, product of gypsum, containing calcium sulphate, used with water, forming a hard case when dry.

Can be obtained loose or already rubbed into muslin as Cellona bandages.

Plaster bandages are generally 4 to 6 yd. long and 3 to 8 in. wide. They should be stored in airtight tins.

Trolley for Application of Plaster of Paris:

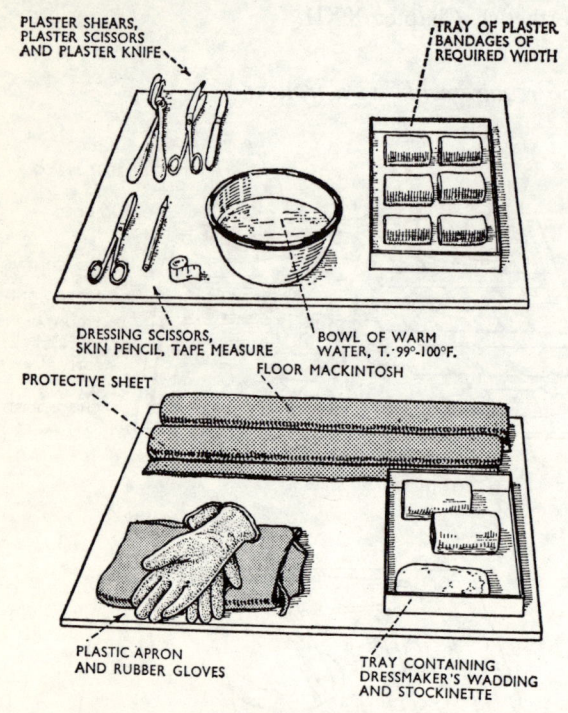

Fig. 73
Trolley for application of plaster of Paris.

Applying plaster

1. Position patient.
2. Apply padding or stockinette to part.

3. Place bandage in water until bubbles cease to rise, lift carefully with both hands and compress gently, loosen free end and hand to surgeon.
4. Place next bandage in water.
5. Each bandage is applied quickly and evenly, moulded to shape of part, special attention given to prominences, and to parts subject to strain which may require reinforcing.
6. Figure of eight turns are avoided.
7. Bandages are smoothed with flat of hand as applied.
8. Appliances such as Bohler's walking iron, heels, wire, rubber tubing, etc., may be incorporated.
9. When bandages are sufficiently thick and plaster has set lightly, it is trimmed with a sharp knife, and if necessary windows are cut. Trimming is performed to allow movement of joints, just beyond the plaster.

Drying of plaster

1. Plaster is marked with date of application and any necessary instructions.
2. With plaster supported on pillows where necessary, the patient is carefully transported to a warm bed, which has fracture boards in position.
3. Protect bed with extra protective and draw sheet where necessary.
4. Place inside blanket next to patient, leaving plaster uncovered and perineal towel in position if required.
5. Cover with cradle and replace bedclothes, turning bottom back over cradle, leaving end of bed open to allow air to circulate and moisture to escape.
6. Carefully turn patient at four-hourly intervals to allow both sides of plaster to dry.
7. Watch carefully for (*a*) denting of plaster over heel (*b*) denting of plaster when bedpan is used.
8. Allow forty-eight hours for large plaster to dry before weight is applied to it.

Tightness of plaster may cause

1. Swelling.
2. Blueness or pallor.
3. Tingling or numbness.
4. Coldness or pain.

} of extremeties.

It is most important to note these signs for they indicate interference with blood or nerve supply.

Elevate part and inform doctor. If condition is not improved within 20 to 30 minutes, doctor may order plaster to be split or, as it is called, 'bi-valved'.

Out-patients who have had plaster applied should be given written instructions to return at once should any of these signs appear.

PLASTER SLABS are made by folding a bandage when wet into layers one on top of the other.

PLASTER BEDS ARE USED FOR:

1. Tuberculosis of spine (Pott's disease).
2. Following spine-grafting operations.
3. Fracture of spine with paraplegia.
4. Abdominal paralysis in anterior poliomyelitis.
5. Scoliosis (lateral curvature of spine).

ANTERIOR SHELLS ARE USED FOR:

1. Turning cases with tuberculosis of spine.
2. Paraplegic cases.

PLASTER CASTS ARE USED TO:

1. Record deformity.
2. Make appliances for correcting deformity.

SPLINTS

Used for immobilisation and support of an injured part, to correct or prevent deformity, or for protection.

1. External splints

Still very useful in first-aid. May be:

(a) Metal, either firm such as Thomas', or malleable such as Cramer wire.
(b) Wood. Straight, curved, angular, Gooch's.
(c) Poroplastic felt.
(d) Strapping.
(e) Bandages, *e.g.* clavicle, jaw.
(f) Slings.
(g) Plaster of Paris.

2. Internal splints

May take form of:

(a) Metal plate.
(b) Metal pin or screw, *e.g.* neck of femur.
(c) Bone graft, *e.g.* spine. Bone peg.
(d) Silver wire, *e.g.* jaw.
(e) Kangaroo tendon, *e.g.* patella.
(f) Intramedullary nails, *e.g.* shafts of long bones.

PADDING OF EXTERNAL SPLINTS:

1. *Temporary.*—Cotton wool and cotton bandage, adhesive padding or latex.
2. *Permanent.*

Requirements on a tray:

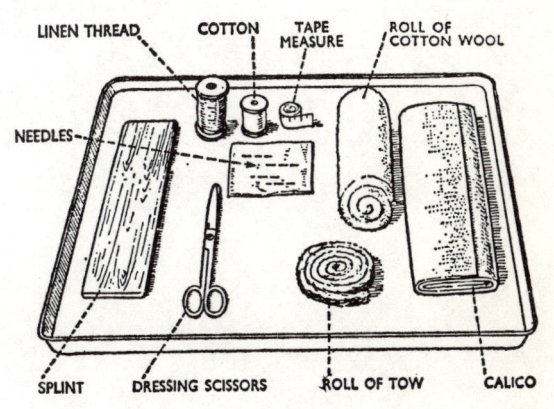

FIG. 74
Tray for padding of external splints.

Method:

1. Cut calico three times width of splint and 6 in. longer.
2. Tease enough tow to make thick springy pad.
3. Place piece of cotton wool ½ inch bigger all round than splint, on calico.
4. Place tow on top of this, fold sides to middle and stitch.
5. Put pad on splint seam side down, and attach using linen thread, taking stitches backwards and forwards across the back of the splint, pulling very tightly.

6. Commence 3 in. from end of splint and finish 3 in. from other end.
7. Make bar of thread at each end by taking several horizontal stitches across back of splint and buttonholing it.
8. Turn in the open ends of calico and attach by thread to cross bars.

Chapter Fourteen

CATHETERISATION

Female and male

FOR FEMALE PATIENT

Explain procedure to patient and screen bed.

It is advisable that the vulva and surrounding parts should be thoroughly washed with soap and water and dried before catheterisation takes place. This can be done by one nurse while second nurse prepares trolley as follows:

Don mask and wash hands.

Mop trolley with Chlorhexidine 0·5 per cent in 70 per cent spirit.

Requirements on a trolley:

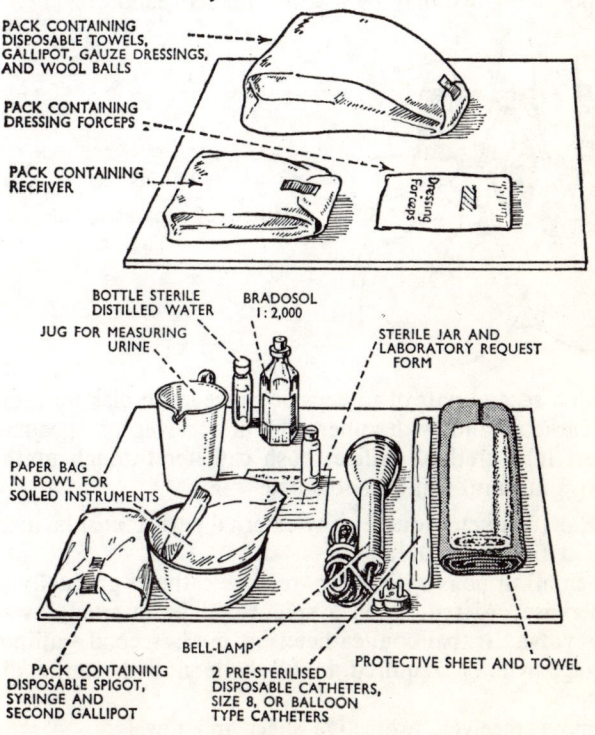

Fig. 75

Trolley for catheterisation of female patient.

PRACTICAL NOTES ON NURSING PROCEDURES

Method:

1. Turn bedclothes back to level of knees and cover patient with blanket.
2. With patient in dorsal position, roll up nightdress, and place protective sheet and towel under buttocks. Place light in position if necessary.
3. Wash and dry hands.
4. Open pack, pour lotion into bowl, tip out instruments, catheters and spigot onto sterile field, place receiver on bed between patient's legs with specimen jar standing in it if necessary.
5. Place sterile towel over abdomen and second one over patient's right thigh.
6. Swab vulva, using forceps in right hand and using fingers of left hand, on swabs, to separate labia. (Once separated labia must be held apart.) Each swab should be used once only, swabbing from front to back of vulva. Discard forceps. A disposable glove may be used on the left hand.

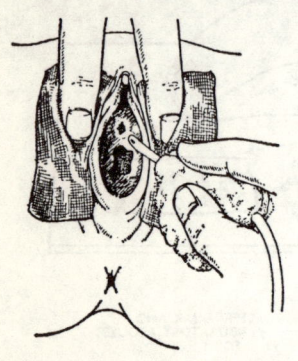

Fig. 76

Method of separating labia.

7. With a second pair of forceps *or* gauze swab pick up eyelet end of catheter and with other end in receiver or specimen jar, insert into urethral orifice; push catheter through urethra for 2 to 3 in. until urine is obtained.

    N.B.—If catheter touches any external part it *must* be discarded and a fresh one used.

8. When all urine is withdrawn, remove catheter gradually (unless otherwise ordered, when a spigot will be inserted), swab and dry vulva. If balloon catheter is used, second gallipot and syringe will be required to fill balloon with sterile distilled water.
9. Remove receiver, protective sheet and towels.
10. Make patient comfortable.
11. Clear away screens and trolleys. Measure and record amount

CATHETERISATION

of urine. Arrange for specimen to go to laboratory with appropriate form, if necessary.

FOR MALE PATIENT

A female nurse is not usually required to assist in the catheterisation of a male patient, unless a female doctor is carrying out the procedure, or the patient is unco-operative and no male assistance is available.

Preparation of trolley:

Don mask and wash hands.

Mop trolley with Chlorhexidine 0·5 per cent in 70 per cent spirit.

Requirements on a trolley:

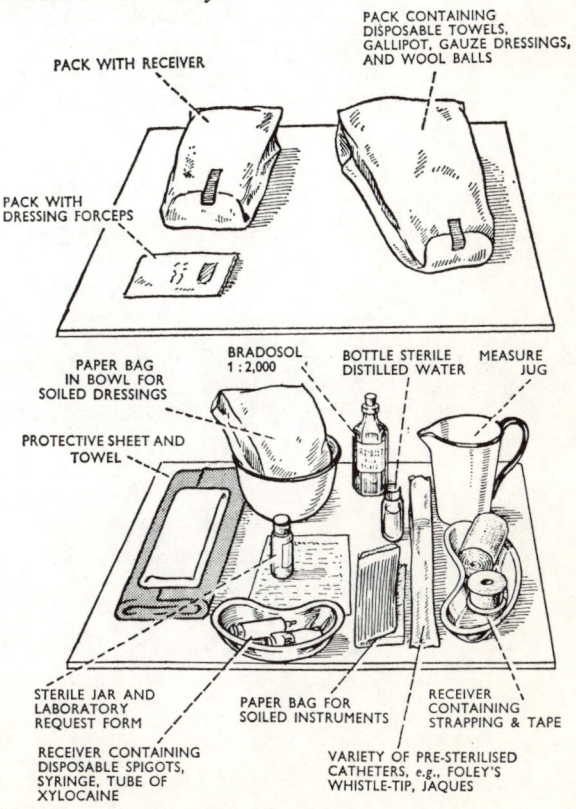

FIG. 77
Trolley for catheterisation of male patient.

Method:

1. Explain procedure to patient and screen bed.
2. Turn bedclothes back to knees and cover patient with blanket.
3. Remove pyjama trousers and leave patient covered and lying in semi-recumbent position.
4. Place trolley in convenient position for doctor.

Chapter Fifteen

VARIETIES OF WASHOUT PROCEDURES

Bladder washout and drainage—Rectal and colostomy washout—Vaginal douching—Insertion of pessaries—Stomach washout—Gastric aspiration

BLADDER WASHOUT

Catheterisation as in Chapter Fourteen.

Additional requirements:
For female patient:

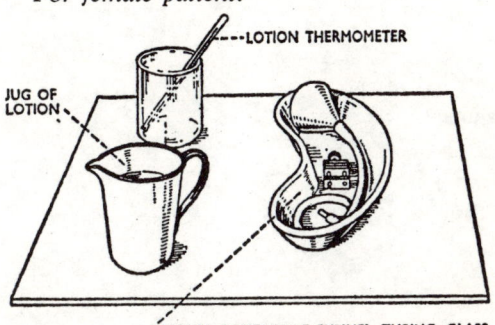

FIG. 78
Trolley for bladder washout, female patient.

Method:

After inserting catheter and expelling air from apparatus, only a small quantity of fluid should be passed into bladder each time, *e.g.* 10 oz, and siphoned back. Process should be repeated until fluid is returned clear. Temperature of lotion 37·8° to 40·6° C (100° to 105° F).

For male patient:

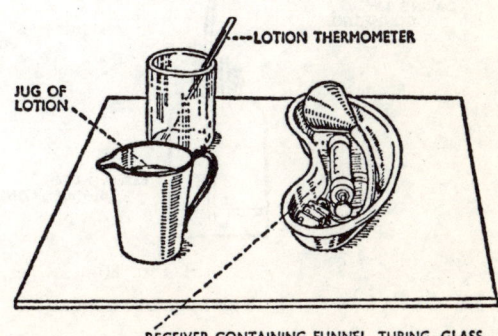

FIG. 79
Trolley for bladder washout, male patient.

Method:

A tube and funnel is generally used for a male bladder washout in which case, after expelling air from apparatus, up to 10 oz of fluid should be put into bladder before siphoning back and great care taken that pressure is not used.

In some cases, *e.g.* after prostatectomy, it is considered advisable to use a bladder syringe, when only 2 to 3 oz of fluid should be inserted at a time.

Tidal drainage

Method employed to combine frequent irrigation and regular emptying of bladder, so that it is kept clean and tone of muscular wall maintained.

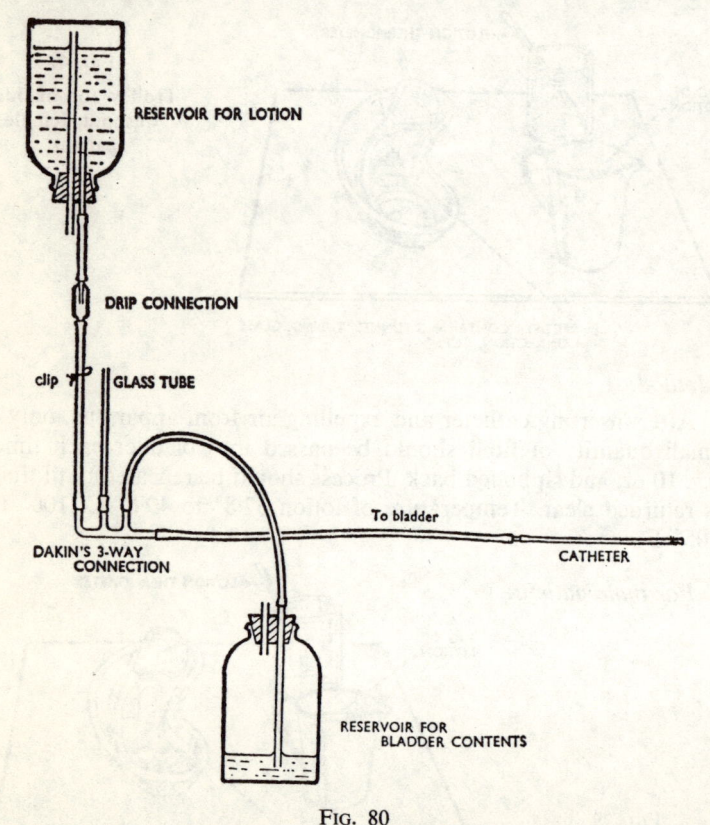

FIG. 80
Tidal dainage apparatus.

N.B.—Plastic bags may be used in place of bottles.

VARIETIES OF WASHOUT PROCEDURES 151

RECTAL WASHOUT

Requirements on a trolley:

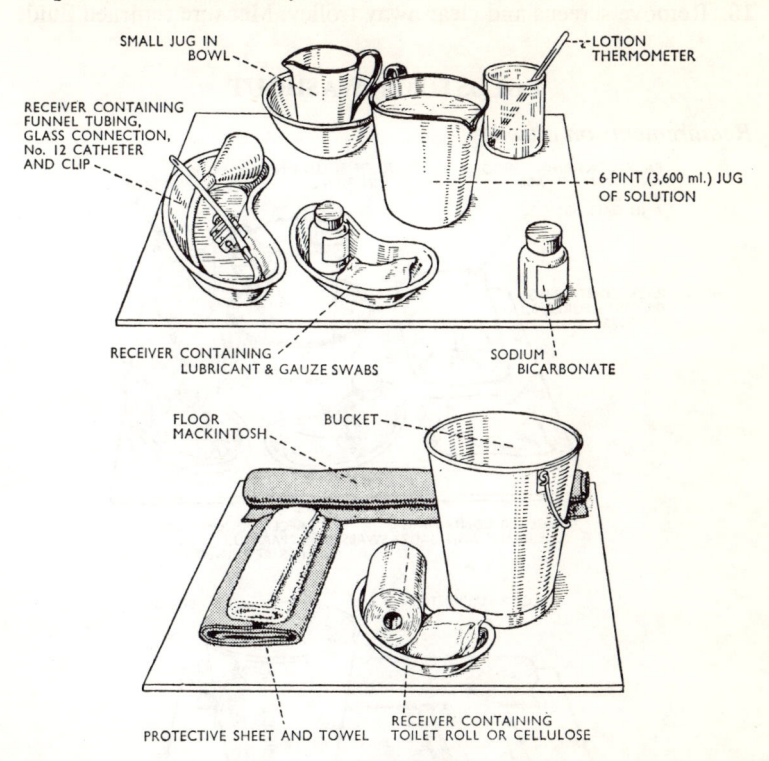

FIG. 81
Trolley for rectal washout.

Method:

1. Explain procedure to patient, screen bed, take trolley to bedside.
2. Prepare patient as for enema. (See Administration of Enemata, Chapter Six.)
3. Place bucket and mackintosh in convenient position on floor.
4. Lubricate catheter and expel air from apparatus by running fluid through; clip tube.
5. Insert catheter through anus into rectum for 3 to 4 in.
6. Release clip and pour in 10 to 20 oz of lotion. Lower funnel, then invert over bucket before completely empty and siphon back fluid.
7. Repeat procedure until fluid returns clear.

8. Remove catheter and wipe anal area with cellulose.
9. Remove protective sheet and towel and make patient comfortable.
10. Remove screens and clear away trolley. Measure returned fluid.

COLOSTOMY WASHOUT

Requirements on a trolley:

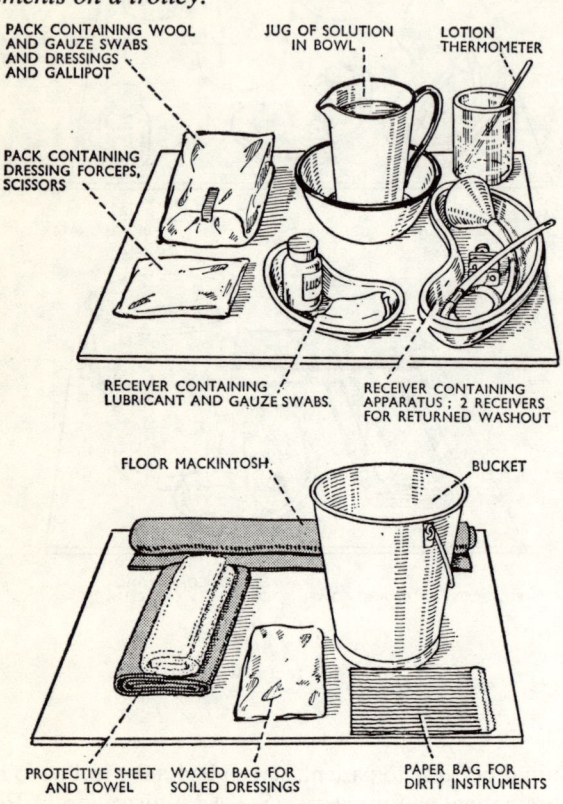

FIG. 82

Trolley for colostomy washout.

VARIETIES OF WASHOUT PROCEDURES

Method:

1. Explain procedure to patient, screen bed and close windows.
2. Turn bedclothes down to pubic area, cover patient's chest with blanket. Turn patient slightly to left side and remove bandage.
3. Place protective sheet in position to protect bedclothes.
4. Wash hands and remove soiled dressing; place receiver in convenient position under colostomy.
5. Lubricate catheter and expel air from apparatus as for enema.
6. Insert catheter into colostomy for about 2 in. and pour in required amount of solution, usually 1 pint.
7. Remove catheter and allow colostomy to act into receiver. Supply patient with second receiver to direct flow of returned fluid.
8. When ready, remove receiver, clean colostomy and surrounding skin. Re-dress, protecting skin, *e.g.* with petroleum jelly gauze and bandage. A Translet colostomy set with disposable bag could be used.
9. Make patient comfortable.
10. Clear away equipment and screens and open windows.

[VAGINAL DOUCHING

VAGINAL DOUCHING

Douche is the term used to describe the washing out of the various cavities of the body, *e.g.* uterus, vagina, ear and nose.

Vaginal douching is used occasionally in treatment of cases where there is discharge from vagina, inflammation of pelvis or local haemorrhage. It may also be used in preparation and after treatment of certain pelvic operations or for persons wearing pessaries.

Requirements on a trolley:

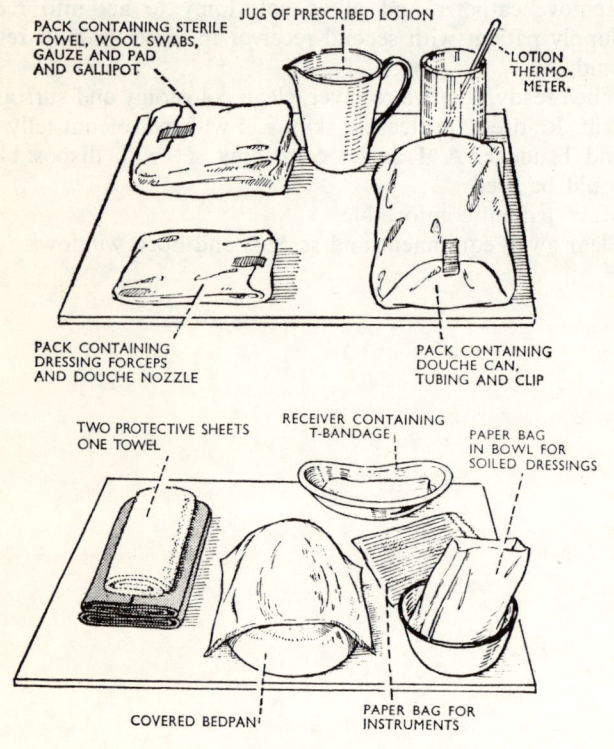

FIG. 83
Trolley for vaginal douching.

Method:

Gown and gloves are worn by nurse if infectious case.
1. Explain procedure to patient.
2. Screen bed and shut windows if necessary.
3. Turn bedclothes down to knees, see that gown is rolled up to

VARIETIES OF WASHOUT PROCEDURES

waist, patient in dorsal position, knees flexed. Cover chest with blanket.
4. Place protective sheet and towel under buttocks, other protective sheet over top bedblothes.
5. Insert warmed bedpan.
6. Wash hands. Place sterile paper towel over top protective sheet.
7. Swab vulva from above downwards, using swab once only, as in catheterisation.
8. Assemble apparatus and expel air by running through fluid.
9. Separate labia and insert douche nozzle gently into vagina, upwards and backwards for about 3 in.
10. Allow fluid to run in, holding can about 1 foot above patient.
11. When can is nearly empty, remove nozzle from vagina, disconnect and place in receiver putting remainder of apparatus in tray.
12. If possible sit patient up and ask her to cough; this helps to expel any remaining fluid.
13. Bedpan is then removed and covered, patient's vulva swabbed and dried. Place pad in position if required.
14. Remove protective sheets and towels. Make patient comfortable and replace bedclothes.
15. Remove and clear away trolley. Inspect bedpan before emptying.
16. Remove screens and open windows.

Points to remember

1. Nurse's hands must be surgically clean.
2. Apparatus must be sterile. Rigid aseptic precautions for postoperative and obstetric cases.
3. Douching lotion must be correct strength and temperature, tested with a thermometer.
4. Vulval orifice must be swabbed.
5. Bed should be protected with protective sheets.

Temperatures used

37·8° to 41·1° C (100° to 106° F) for antiseptic purposes.
43·3° to 46·1° C (110° to 115° F) for inflammation and haemorrhage.

IRRIGATION AND INSERTION OF PESSARIES

Vaginal irrigation is sometimes used after injury or operation on the vagina or perineum.

Requirements as for douching, but a rubber catheter No. 12 or 14 is used instead of a nozzle and a funnel is substituted for the douche can.

The insertion of pessaries

Pessaries are instruments introduced into the vagina to support a displaced uterus in the correct position, *e.g.* in elderly women with a prolapsed uterus or in the treatment of a retroverted uterus.

PESSARIES MAY BE MADE OF:

1. Vulcanite, metal or plastic, rigid type, *e.g.* Hodges.
2. Rubber covered watch-spring, flexible type.

Vulcanite are immersed in antiseptic for sterilisation. Metal, plastic and rubber may be boiled.

Daily douching is necessary when a pessary is worn and it should be removed and cleaned or a new one fitted at least every three months. They are usually inserted by a doctor.

N.B.—Prepacked sterilised plastic pessaries are usually used nowadays.

Medicated pessaries are small tablets or gelatinous substances containing medicaments which are introduced into the vagina in the treatment of inflammatory conditions, *e.g.* vaginitis.

Use and insertion of tampons

Vaginal tampons are used in treatment of inflammatory conditions of the genital tract or to control haemorrhage from the uterus or vagina. They can be made of cotton wool covered by gauze with a tape attached to facilitate removal. A vaginal douche is usually given before the insertion of a tampon.

The bladder must be emptied before insertion which is usually carried out at night and tampon removed in morning.

VARIETIES OF WASHOUT PROCEDURES

Requirements on a tray:

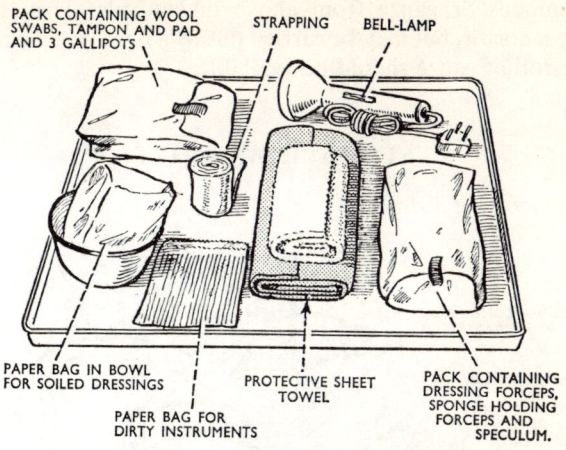

FIG. 84
Tray for insertion of tampons.

An Anglepoise lamp is often used now, instead of a bell-lamp.

Method:

1. Explain procedure to patient and screen bed.
2. Turn bedclothes down to knees and cover top of patient with blanket.
3. Place patient in left lateral or dorsal position with protective sheet and towel under buttocks.
4. Place lamp in position to give good light.
5. Wash hands and put on gloves.
6. Swab vulva.
7. Lubricate and insert speculum by passing over perineum on to posterior wall of vagina and gently pushing upwards and backwards.
8. Tampon soaked in the medicament is then grasped with sponge-holding forceps and passed well up to cervix, speculum being gradually withdrawn.
9. Tape is then strapped to patient's thigh, and clean pad placed in position.
10. Remove gloves.
11. Remove protective sheet and towel and make patient comfortable. Remake bed.
12. Remove tray and screens. Clear away equipment.

If tampon is used to control haemorrhage, entire vagina is plugged with tampons or gauze from above downwards. This is usually done by a doctor, but may be carried out by a nurse in an emergency. A large roll of gauze should be available.

STOMACH WASHOUT

Requirements on a trolley:

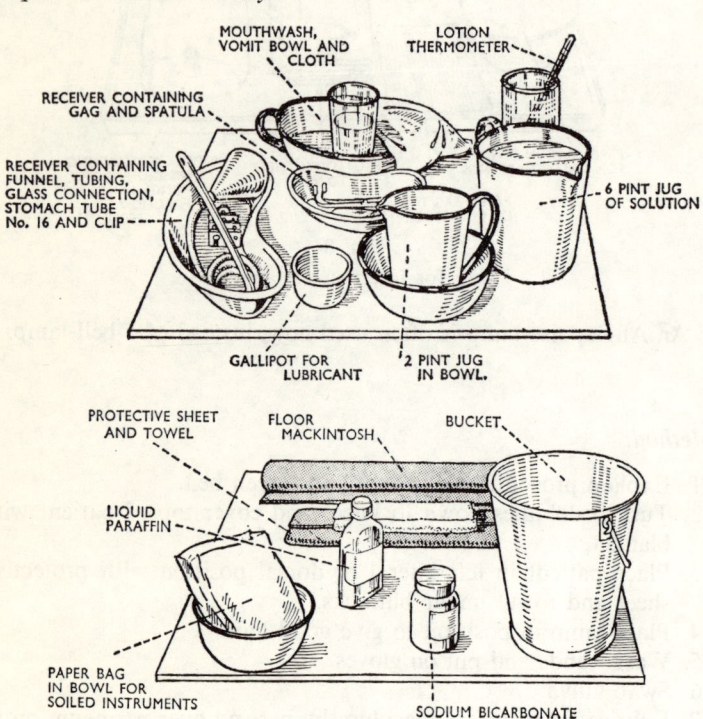

FIG. 85
Trolley for stomach washout.

Method:

1. Explain procedure to patient and screen bed.
2. Place floor mackintosh in position with bucket standing on it.
3. If possible, sit patient well up and place protective sheet and towel round neck and over bedclothes. Remove dentures and place in mug of water.
4. Lubricate stomach tube and pass well back over tongue into pharynx and oesophagus without touching back of throat if

VARIETIES OF WASHOUT PROCEDURES

possible. Tell patient to breathe deeply all the time, and to swallow frequently to aid passage of tube.

N.B.—If patient becomes cyanosed or coughs, tube should be withdrawn and re-passed.

A gag and tongue depressor may be used for an unconscious patient, who should be in a semi-recumbent position with head turned to one side.

This procedure may be done in annexe or bathroom, if patient's condition allows.

5. Attach funnel to tube and lower to below stomach level to allow escape of gas and stomach contents. Tube is then clipped before raising to level of chin, to prevent air entry.
6. Fill funnel with solution, undo clip and allow ½ pint to run in, then lower funnel, before completely empty, over bucket to siphon fluid back.
7. Repeat process until fluid returns clear. (Discontinue if blood appears, pain is complained of, or patient is exhausted.)
8. Clip tube, withdraw evenly and quickly and place in receiver.
9. Give patient mouthwash; clean dentures. Make comfortable.
10. Remove screens. Clear equipment, measure returned fluid and record character.

INTERMITTENT GASTRIC ASPIRATION

Requirements on a tray:

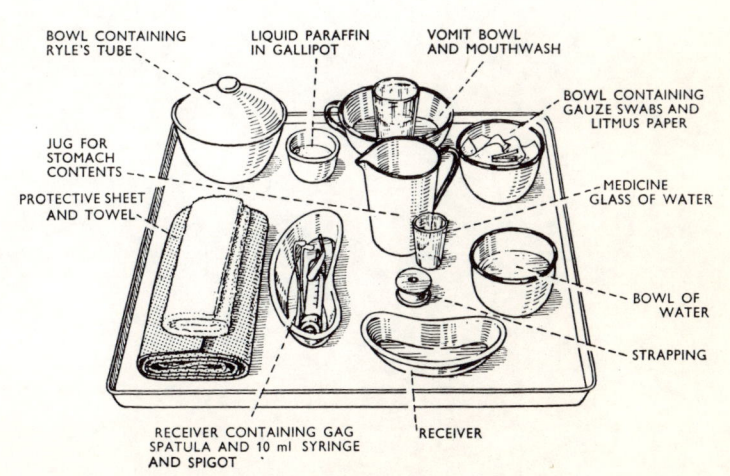

FIG. 86

Tray for intermittent gastric aspiration.

Method:

1. Explain procedure to patient and screen bed.
2. Protect patient's gown and bedclothes with protective sheet and towel.
3. Lubricate Ryle's tube and pass through nose or mouth (nose must be cleaned first if this route is used) as for stomach tube.
4. Attach syringe and withdraw fluid, place in jug and test with litmus paper. Rinse syringe.
5. Spigot tube, strap to patient's cheek with small piece of strapping.
6. Measure aspirated fluid and record.
7. Repeat aspiration at regular intervals as ordered by doctor.

Patient will require frequent attention to mouth either cleaning or mouthwashes according to condition.

If treatment is carried out for more than twenty-four hours, tray must be re-set each morning with fresh equipment.

Ryle's tube is changed every 2 to 3 days.

CONTINUOUS GASTRIC ASPIRATION

Method used when stomach requires to be kept continuously empty. Apparatus attached to Ryle's tube after passing as for intermittent gastric aspiration. Suction maintained by reversing water reservoirs as necessary.

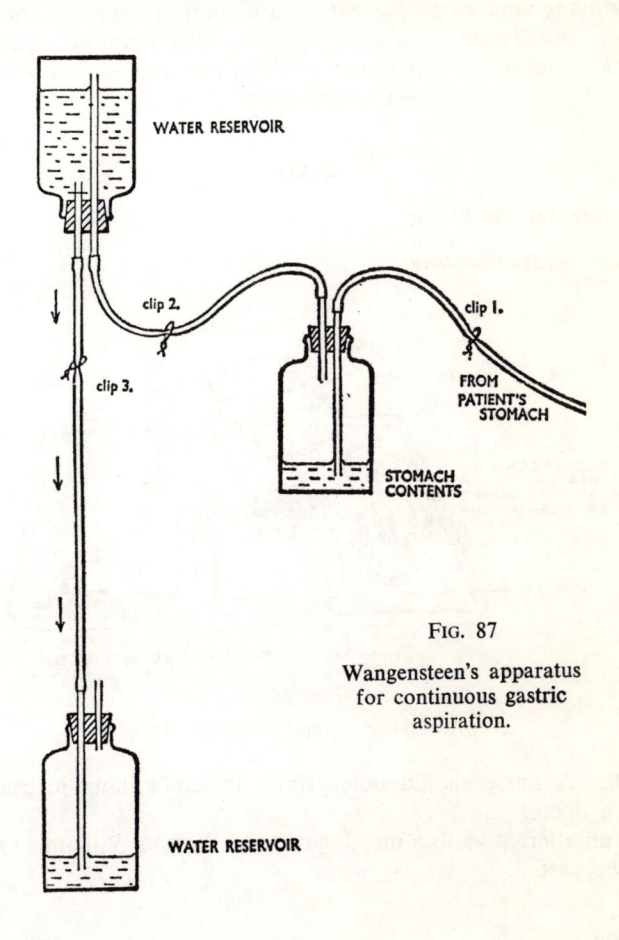

FIG. 87

Wangensteen's apparatus for continuous gastric aspiration.

Chapter Sixteen

EAR, NOSE AND THROAT TREATMENTS

Syringing, and swabbing ear—Instillation of drops—Cleaning nose, instillation of drops—Spraying and painting throat—Tracheotomy — Antrostomy — Myringotomy — Peritonsillar abscess—Control of nasal bleeding

EAR

Syringing and swabbing

Requirements on a tray:

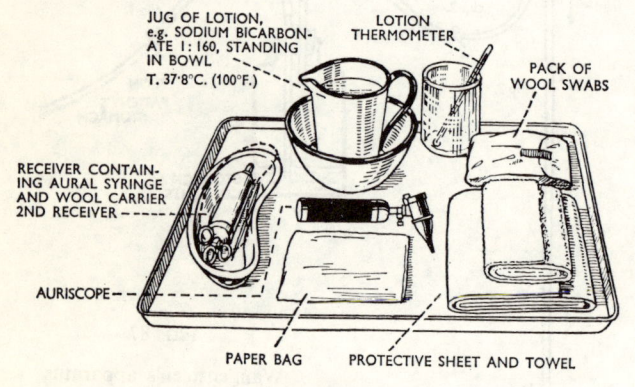

Fig. 88
Tray for syringing and swabbing the ear.

N.B.—A nurse should not syringe an ear without instructions from a doctor.

As an alternative to a metal syringe, a Watson William's syringe may be used.

Method:

1. Sit patient on a chair in a good light; if in bed, prop upright on pillows. Place protective sheet and towel round shoulders.
2. Give patient receiver to hold under ear. Look into meatus using auriscope, to ascertain what has to be removed.
3. Fill syringe with lotion and expel air by pressing lightly on

piston with syringe held upright. The temperature of lotion should be 37·8° C (100° F).
4. To straighten meatus, gently pull pinna of ear upwards and backwards, with left hand and then, with syringe in right hand direct flow of lotion along roof of canal. Repeat as necessary.
5. When irrigation is completed, remove receiver and gently swab out meatus by securely winding wool on to wool carrier, leaving a loose tuft at the end. Look into meatus to make sure it is clear.
6. Remove protective sheet from patient's shoulders.
7. Clear away tray. Boil nozzle of syringe together with equipment. Dry and put away.

Instillation of drops

Requirements on a tray:

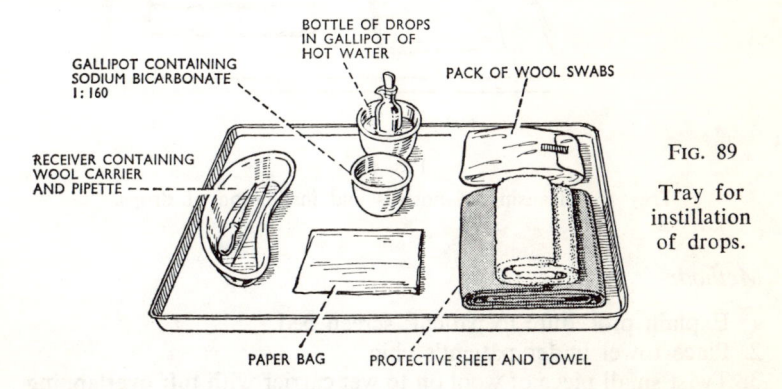

FIG. 89

Tray for instillation of drops.

Method:

1. Place patient in comfortable convenient position. Place protective sheet and towel round shoulder.
2. Mop out ear gently, using wool on carrier and sodium bicarbonate solution, and dry.
3. Instil 2 or 3 drops into meatus with pipette, holding pinna upwards and backwards to straighten canal.
4. Instruct patient to keep ear uppermost for few minutes. Massage gently, just in front of entrance to meatus to achieve good penetration of drops.
5. Dry entrance to pinna. Remove protective sheet and towel. Clear away equipment.

Powder, *e.g.* sulphathiazole, may sometimes be ordered to dry up the skin of the external auditory meatus. This is blown into the canal with an insufflator.

NOSE

Cleansing the nostrils and instillation of drops

Requirements on a tray:

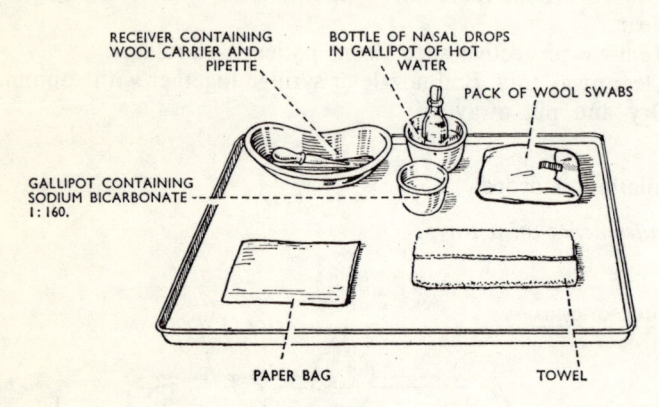

FIG. 90
Tray for cleansing of nostrils and instillation of drops.

Method:

1. Explain procedure to patient; screen bed.
2. Place towel under patient's chin.
3. Twist small piece of wool on to wet carrier with tuft overlapping end. Dip in sodium bicarbonate solution and gently clean nostril. If patient able to do so, may clean own nose by blowing gently, first one side then other.
4. Repeat as often as necessary, removing soiled wool with dissecting forceps.
5. To instil drops, ask patient to tip head backwards and with pipette drop 2 or 3 drops into each nostril, head being slightly tilted to appropriate side and opposite nostril being compressed.
6. Patient should breathe through mouth and be asked to keep head tilted back for few minutes before being made comfortable.
7. Clear away equipment.

Nasal washouts or douching

The patient sniffs normal saline solution through each nostril separately into pharynx and then spits it out together with any muco-purulent material from the nose.

Douching of the nose with a pressure syringe is dangerous because infection may be carried along Eustachian tube to middle ear.

THROAT

Spraying, painting and gargling

Requirements on a tray:

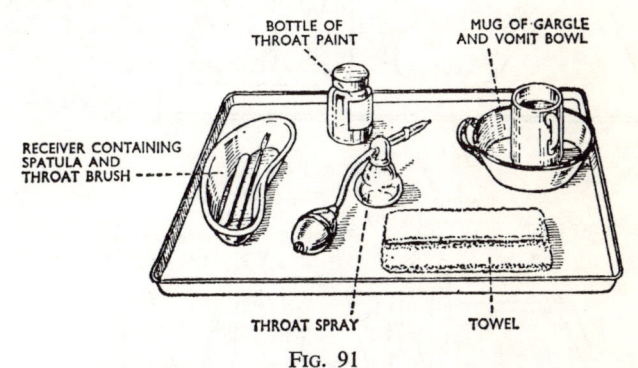

FIG. 91
Tray for spraying, painting, and gargling throat.

Gargling

A towel is placed under the patient's chin and the patient instructed to take small mouthfuls of gargle and with head back hold fluid at back of throat and force air up through it.

Spraying

The patient opens the mouth while the nurse passes the nozzle of the spray over the tongue and then squeezes the bulb, when a spray will be directed on to the throat.

Painting

After gargling, patient opens mouth while nurse with brush dipped in Mandl's paint, and holding tongue down with a spatula, gently applies it to sides of throat, being careful not to touch soft palate or back of pharynx or patient will retch.

TRACHEOTOMY

Requirements on a trolley:

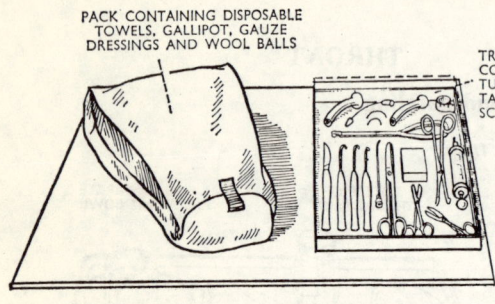

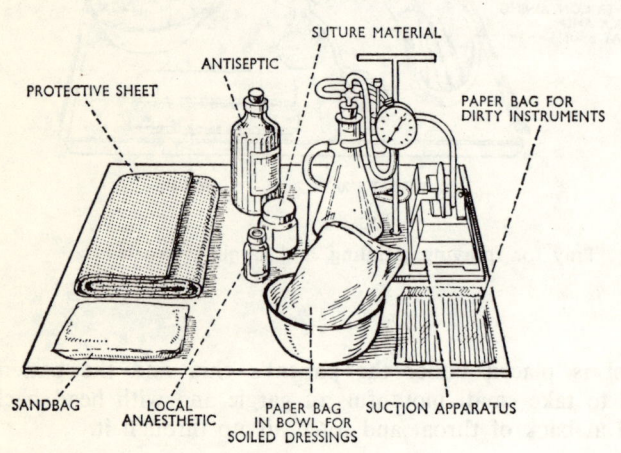

Fig. 92
Tray for tracheotomy.

POSITION OF PATIENT.—Recumbent with shoulders slightly raised on pillows. Sandbag placed under the shoulders to extend the head which must be held exactly in the midline.

AFTERCARE.—Patient is returned to a warmed bed and placed in semi-recumbent or sitting position, unless contra-indicated.

The patient must have a special nurse in attendance day and night for 4 to 5 days at least.

EAR, NOSE AND THROAT TREATMENTS

Requirements on a trolley:

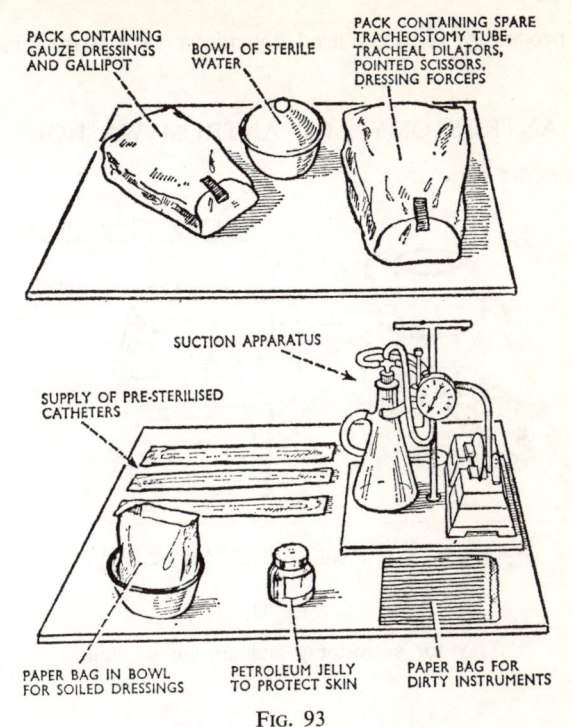

FIG. 93

Tray for after-care of tracheotomy.

Suction apparatus should be used regularly to keep the tube clear. Each hour the inner tube should be removed and washed in sodium bicarbonate solution and then replaced. Dressings must be changed frequently as they become soiled.

The nurse must see that the airway is kept clear. Secretion coughed up should be gently wiped away to prevent it being sucked back into tube.

The outer tube is changed only by the surgeon except when it is coughed out. In event of this happening the nurse must quickly put dilator into opening and then introduce spare outer tube and secure it with tapes round the neck.

A writing pad and pencil must be provided for patient who will be voiceless.

When patient is left for short periods a bell must be placed within easy reach.

Intubation

This procedure is rarely used nowadays. (See Appendix.)

ANTROSTOMY AND ANTRUM WASHOUT

Requirements on a tray:

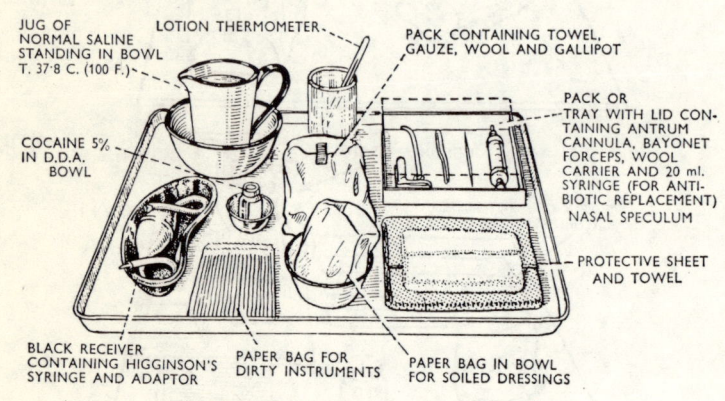

Fig. 94

Tray for antrostomy and antrum washout.

MYRINGOTOMY

Requirements on a tray:

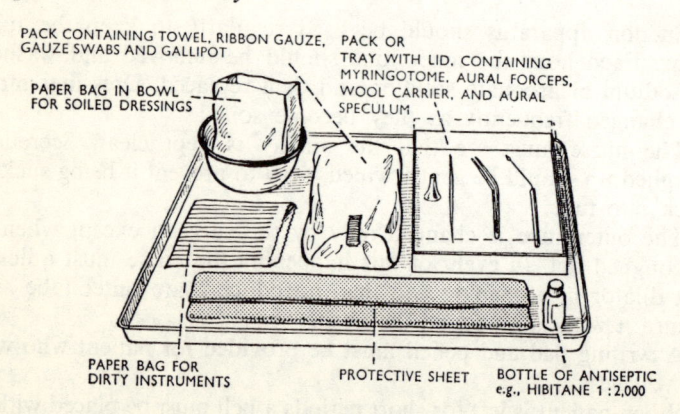

Fig. 95

Tray for myringotomy.

EAR, NOSE AND THROAT TREATMENTS

In addition, general anaesthetic equipment will be required, also mirror and light or auriscope.

A pad and bandage may also be required.

OPENING OF PERI-TONSILLAR ABSCESS

Requirements on a tray:

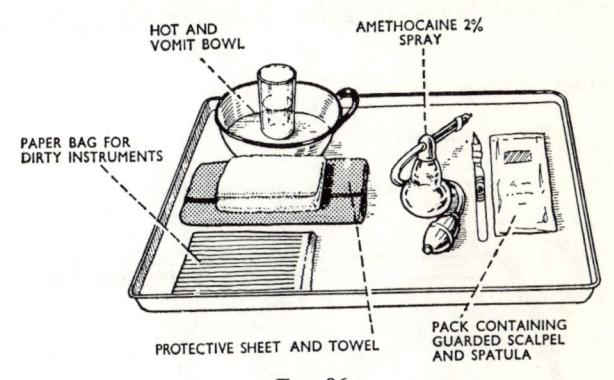

FIG. 96
Tray for opening of peri-tonsillar abscess.

For children, a general anaesthetic is required.
N.B. Guarded scalpel shown on tray would be in pack.

CONTROL OF NASAL BLEEDING

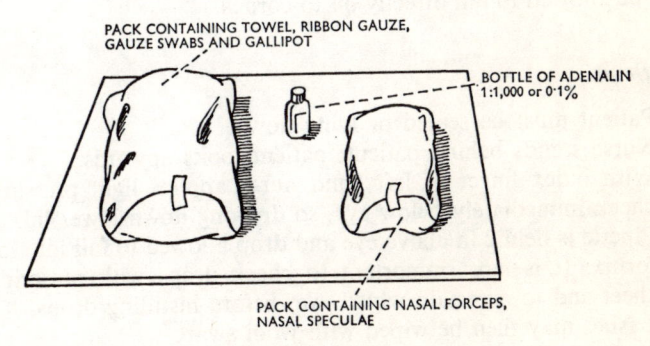

FIG. 97
Tray for packing nasal cavities.

Chapter Seventeen

EYE TREATMENTS

Instillation of drops—Swabbing, spoon bathing and irrigation

Instillation of drops

Requirements on a tray:

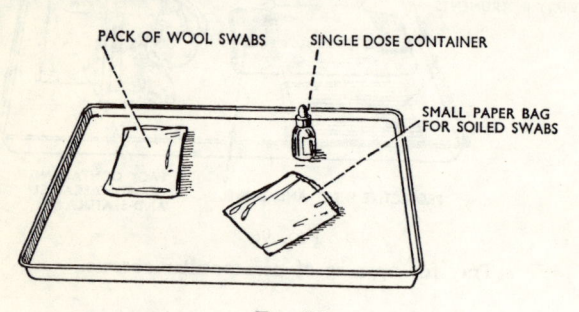

FIG. 98
Tray for instillation of eye drops.

This procedure should be carried out very gently and drops must not be allowed to fall directly on to cornea.

Method:

1. Patient must be seated or lying down.
2. Nurse stands behind patient; patient looks upwards.
3. With index finger of left hand nurse applies light pressure to cheek immediately below eye, so drawing down lower lid.
4. Pipette is held 2 in above eye and drop allowed to fall into lower fornix. It is most important to check drops with prescription sheet and to ascertain which eye, before instilling drops.
5. Lashes may then be wiped with wool swab.

Ointment may be applied to eye either from small collapsible tube with fine opening when lower lid is pulled down and a thin line of ointment squeezed into the lower fornix, or glass rod may be used, keeping it parallel with lid to prevent poking eye.

EYE TREATMENTS 171

Swabbing and spoon bathing
Requirements on a tray:

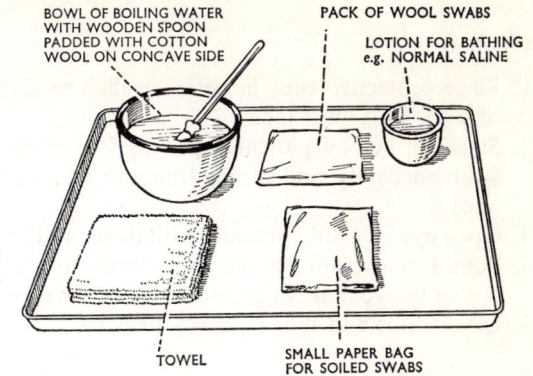

BOWL OF BOILING WATER WITH WOODEN SPOON PADDED WITH COTTON WOOL ON CONCAVE SIDE

PACK OF WOOL SWABS

LOTION FOR BATHING e.g. NORMAL SALINE

TOWEL

SMALL PAPER BAG FOR SOILED SWABS

FIG. 99

Tray for swabbing and spoon bathing.

Method:
1. Place towel around patient's neck.
2. Place tray in front of patient and instruct him to hold padded spoon up to affected eye and allow steam to circulate round closed eye. Spoon is re-dipped into water at frequent intervals.
3. Eye may then be gently swabbed from inner side outwards, using each swab once only.
4. Dry in same way and leave patient comfortable.
5. Clear away tray.

This treatment may be carried out for 15 minutes every 2 hours. It is unwise to go out into a cold atmosphere immediately after this treatment.

Irrigation
Requirements on a tray:

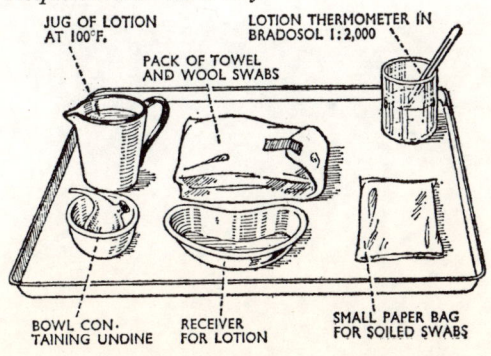

JUG OF LOTION AT 100°F.

LOTION THERMOMETER IN BRADOSOL 1:2,000

PACK OF TOWEL AND WOOL SWABS

BOWL CONTAINING UNDINE

RECEIVER FOR LOTION

SMALL PAPER BAG FOR SOILED SWABS

FIG. 100

Tray for irrigation.

Tray should be placed on trolley with shoulder blanket and protective cape placed on bottom shelf.

Method:

1. Place protective cape in position, then receiver, with large piece of wool to protect face.
2. Standing behind patient wipe lids free of discharge, using each swab once only, and wiping from the inner corner to outer corner of eye.
3. Open eye by gentle pressure with finger and thumb.
4. Pour lotion from undine over cheek first and then into inner corner of eye. Patient is instructed to move eye up and down.
5. Dry eyelids and face with wool swabs.

Chapter Eighteen

ARTIFICIAL FEEDING

Gastrostomy—Jejunostomy—Oesophageal and nasal

Gastrostomy

Gastrostomy means an opening into the stomach through the abdominal wall. It is usually performed when there is a permanent obstruction of the oesophagus. It is usual for a self-retaining catheter to be placed in position for the first week or ten days, until a permanent tract has been made, when an ordinary catheter can be used and the opening closed with a flanged bougie between feeds. The area of skin surrounding the wound should be protected from the irritation and digestive action of the gastric juices.

Requirements on a tray:

JUG CONTAINING NOURISHING FLUID e.g. MILK, MILKY PREPARATION, EGG AND MILK, SOUPS ETC., IN A BOWL OF WARM WATER

WARM STERILE WATER IN MEDICINE GLASS

RECEIVER CONTAINING FUNNEL, TUBING, GLASS CONNECTION, CATHETER (AFTER FIRST WEEK OR TEN DAYS), CLIP, FOOD THERMOMETER

PROTECTIVE SHEET AND TOWEL

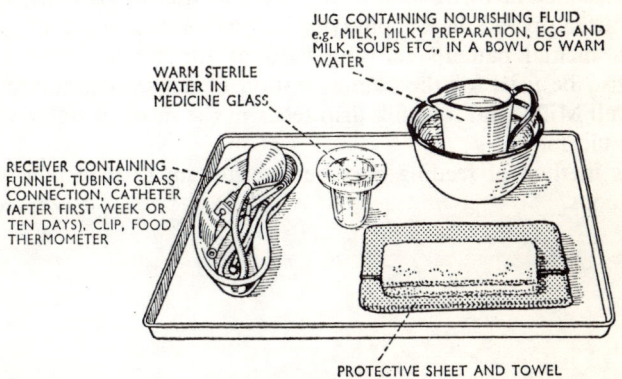

FIG. 101
Tray for gastrostomy.

Method:

1. Explain procedure to patient and screen bed.
2. Place patient in comfortable position and turn bedclothes back as far as necessary to expose area.
3. Place protective sheet and towel in position to protect bed.
4. Expel air from the apparatus and connect tubing to catheter;

run a little water through tube followed by feed and then a little more water to clear tube which is then clipped off.
5. Disconnect tube and funnel.
6. Replace bandage and make patient comfortable.
7. Remove tray and screens.

Patient will require frequent mouthwashes to keep mouth clean and moist.

Jejunostomy feeding

Jejunostomy means an opening into the jejunum, used for feeding in a similar way to the gastrostomy. It is used where the stomach is unable to tolerate any food. Small feeds are needed at more frequent intervals and the food is often predigested. The skin around the opening requires protection with ointment.

Oesophageal and nasal feeding

This may be ordered for cases of paralysis of the soft palate or muscles concerned with swallowing, for unconscious patients, sometimes after operations on pharynx, larynx or trachea, for weakly babies, mental patients refusing food or for 'hunger strikers'. It may also be used for the administration of nauseating substances, *e.g.* 'Bull Milk', and for milk drip feeds in the medical treatment of peptic ulcers.

This method of feeding may be intermittent (2 to 4 hourly) or continuous.

ARTIFICIAL FEEDING 175

Requirements on a trolley:

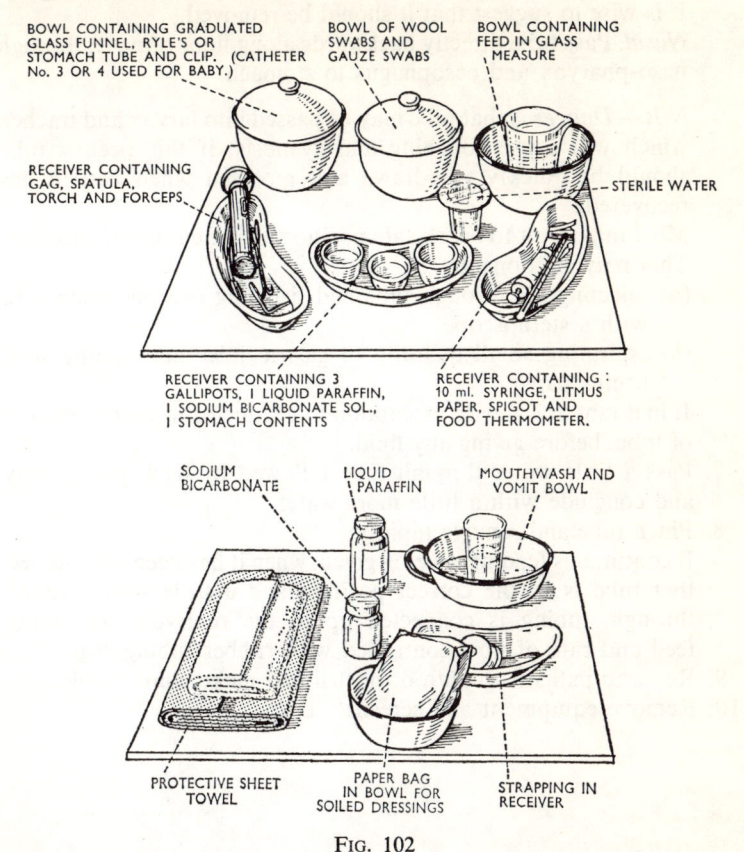

FIG. 102
Trolley for oesophageal and nasal feeding.

Method:

1. Explain procedure to patient and screen bed.
2. Sit patient up if possible, place bib or protective sheet and napkin in position.
3. Wash hands.
4. Swab patient's mouth or nostrils if necessary. If conscious, may clear own nose by blowing into paper tissue.
5. Moisten tube in sterile water or lubricate with glycerine or liquid paraffin.
6. *Oesophageal.* Pass tube towards side of mouth, taking care not to touch sensitive parts, so causing retching. Encourage patient

to swallow during passage of tube. If patient has dental plate, it is wise to suggest that it should be removed.

Nasal. Pass tube directly backwards along floor of nose, through naso-pharynx and oesophagus to stomach.

N.B.—Danger is that tube may be passed into larynx and trachea which will cause coughing and cyanosis; if this occurs, tube should be quickly withdrawn and repassed when patient has recovered.

Most important to check safe position, if patient is unconscious. This may be done by:
- (*a*) injecting air through tube and listening over stomach area with a stethoscope,
- (*b*) aspirating small quantity of gastric juice and testing with litmus paper.

If in doubt, it is a wise precaution to get doctor to check position of tube, before giving any fluid.

7. Pass a little water through tube followed by feed; give slowly and conclude with a little more water.
8. Pinch tube and remove rapidly.

If continuous feeding is being given, when it has been ascertained that tube is in the correct position and a little water passed through, tubing is connected up to the reservoir containing feed and rate of flow controlled with rubber tubing clip.

9. Re-swab patient's mouth or nostril and make comfortable.
10. Remove equipment and screens.

Chapter Nineteen

INFUSIONS

Subcutaneous, intravenous and intramedullary—Blood donors

SUBCUTANEOUS (HYPODERMOCLYSIS)

Intermittent and continuous.

Requirements on a trolley:

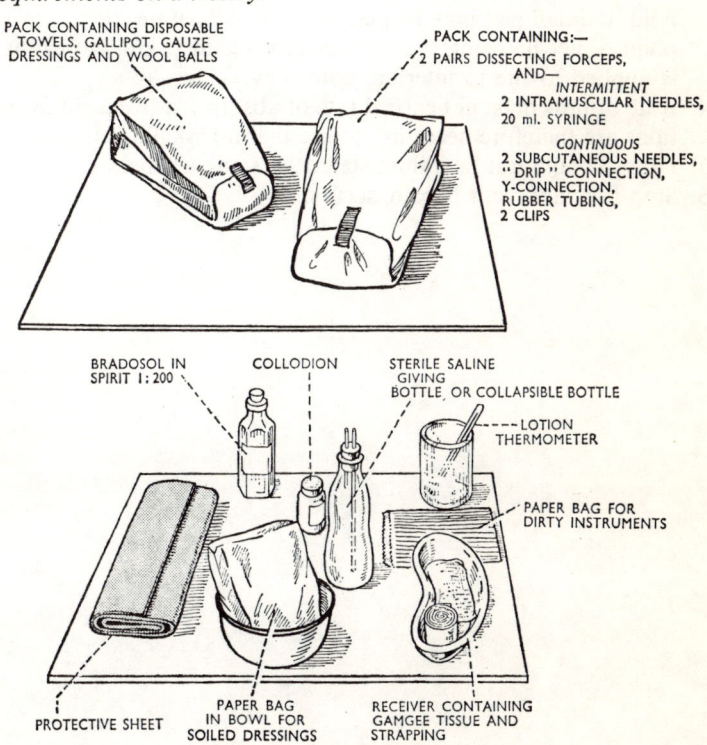

FIG. 103
Trolley for subcutaneous infusions.

Site

1. Lateral chest wall. Needle is inserted behind lower border of

pectoral muscles clear of breast so that fluid goes into loose tissue of axilla.
2. Abdominal wall. Needle is inserted lateral to umbilicus, point directly upwards and outwards.
3. Outer sides of thighs. Needle is inserted mid-way between great trochanter and knee, pointing towards hip.

Technique

1. Strict asepsis must be observed.
2. To aid absorption, hyalase may be injected at the commencement of infusion.
3. Dressing is applied over puncture site and strapping arranged to hold it. Small pad may be placed under butt of needle to prevent point of needle being pressed upwards against skin. No bandage is applied to site to interfere with flow.
4. Rate of flow must not exceed rate of absorption; frequent inspections are therefore necessary to see that no swelling is present.
5. Drugs should not be administered by same needle.
6. Stop flow and wait if pain occurs.

INFUSIONS

INTRAVENOUS

Requirements on a trolley:

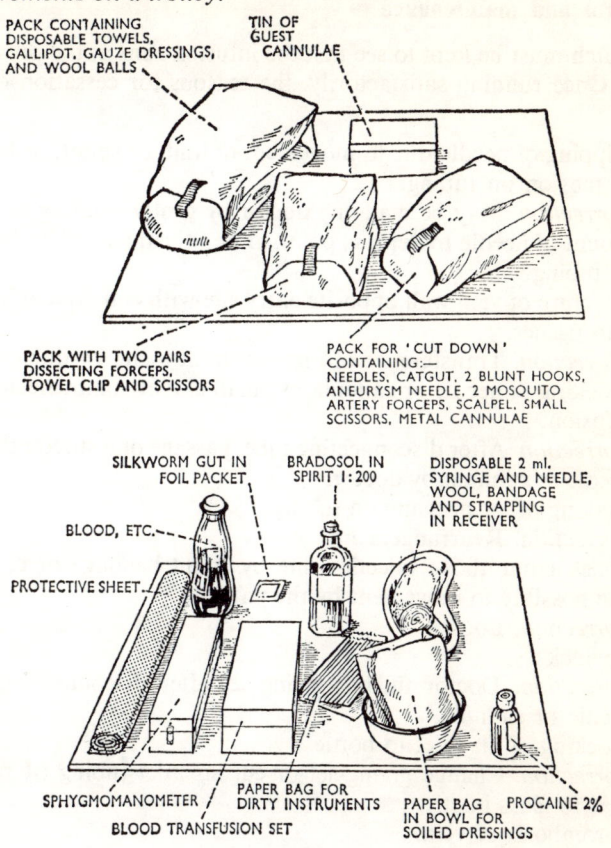

FIG. 104
Trolley for intravenous infusions.

N.B.—Disposable Guest cannulae, 'intra-cath' cannulae and other makes are now available.

Two methods, *e.g.* 'needle' and 'cut down'. In first method sharp needle is inserted through skin into vein and in second, skin incision is made, vein exposed and blunt cannula inserted. There is now a special intravenous needle which introduces very fine polythene tubing into vein.

Important to avoid any pressure on limb. Needle or cannula covered by pad and held in place by netalast or tubegauze, the tubing being looped round fingers to prevent any pull on it.

Control and maintenance

Watch must be kept to see that the infusion runs at the prescribed rate. Once running satisfactorily, the reasons for cessation of flow are:

1. Slipping of needle due to movement of limb or splint, or because of tension on tubing.
   Correction. May be made by doctor by gently rotating or lifting mount of needle to depress point, after adjustment of limb, splint or tubing.
2. Puncture of vein wall opposite entry site with consequent leakage into tissues.
   Correction. Transference of infusion to new site by doctor.
3. Blocking of needle or cannula by small clot at commencement of infusion.
   Correction. After disconnecting tube, passage of a stilette through needle or cannula by doctor.
4. Kinking of, or pressure on tubing.
   Correction. Rearrangement.
5. Constriction above injection site by splint bandage or clothing, due possibly to movement by the patient.
   Correction. Loosen.
6. Air locks.
   Correction. Doctor flushes giving-set after disconnecting from needle or cannula.
7. Blocking of air inlet to bottle.
   Correction. Change giving-set or cut air inlet tubing (if rubber) near to glass inlet.
8. Thrombosis of vein.
   Correction. Infusion transferred to alternative site by doctor.

Observations

Temperature, pulse and respiration should be recorded hourly throughout transfusion and for two hours afterwards. If shock is present, the pulse may be recorded $\frac{1}{4}$ or $\frac{1}{2}$ hourly.

To change bottle

This should be done just before level of fluid reaches bottle neck. The control clip is closed as near needle or cannula as possible. The empty bottle is taken down and placed on locker. The screw cap of the fresh bottle is removed and the bung complete with glass and rubber tubing is transferred from the empty bottle to the new one, care being taken not to contaminate the glass tubes in any way. The new bottle is then inverted (drips from the air inlet being caught in the sterile cap of the bottle), hung up and the control clip opened and rate of flow adjusted.

To discontinue

Close control clip. Place sterile pad over needle or cannula after removal of dressings, press on site of injection and withdraw needle or cannula. The pad is then bandaged firmly in position to prevent leakage.

Complications

General.—Rapid rise of temperature, or rigor.
Increased pulse rate.
Bubbly cough, rising pulse rate, rising respiration rate, indicate excessive fluid intake.
Pain in loin.
Oedema.
Air embolus.

Local.— Thrombosis.
Sepsis.
Haematoma and oedema.

BONE MARROW INFUSION (Intramedullary)

A rare procedure, but of great value in cases of extensive burns where no vein is readily accessible. It may be given into the sternum or subcutaneous surface of the tibia. The chief risk is sepsis and great care is necessary that the technique should be fully aseptic.

Requirements.—As for intravenous infusion with addition of a sternal puncture needle.

BLOOD DONORS AND THE TAKING OF BLOOD

In this country the Ministry of Health runs a Blood Transfusion Service with a national blood bank. The blood is supplied by volunteers. It must be remembered that donors are doing a public service for which they are not paid. They should be treated with respect and gratitude. This procedure is carried out with a standard 'taking-set' which consists of a bung with 2 short glass tubes, rubber tubing and a short bevel needle, *e.g.* French's. The whole is wrapped in cellophane and sterilised in a sealed tin.

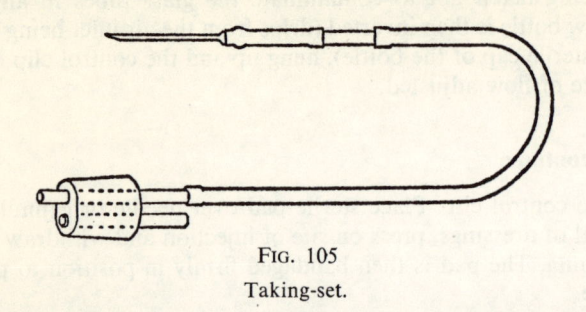

Fig. 105
Taking-set.

500 ml of blood is usually withdrawn from a healthy donor, into a special type of sterile bottle containing anti-coagulant. It is important that the donor's name and address is checked and recorded on the card which accompanies the bottle of blood. It is also important that the blood donor has a medical check. If the history reveals any form of jaundice, then the donor is rejected

The donor must rest for a short time after giving blood.

Chapter Twenty

DRAINAGE AND EXPLORATION OF BODY CAVITIES

Exploration and aspiration of chest—Artificial pneumothorax—Paracentesis abdominis—Southey's tubes—Lumbar puncture

CHEST

EXPLORATION OF CHEST

A simple procedure performed when the presence of fluid in the pleural cavity is suspected. A hollow bore needle of suitable length is introduced through an intercostal space under local anaesthetic. If fluid is found, a small quantity is withdrawn for examination.

ASPIRATION OF CHEST

This is the withdrawal of large quantities of pleural effusion.

After explaining procedure to patient the bed is screened and windows closed if necessary.

The patient may be sat up leaning forward over a bed table on which is placed a pillow, or lying semi-recumbent on unaffected side with arm supported over head. The patient is warned not to cough without first warning doctor.

After the procedure is over the patient is made comfortable and the screens and trolley removed, the windows re-opened.

Alternative apparatus:

1. Syringe with 2-way adaptor.
2. 3-way syringe.
3. Potain's aspirator, rarely used nowadays, as it is thought that fluid is withdrawn too rapidly.
4. Continuous suction apparatus, *e.g.* Wangensteen's bottles or electric pump.
5. Martin's chest aspirator.

184 PRACTICAL NOTES ON NURSING PROCEDURES

Requirements on a trolley:

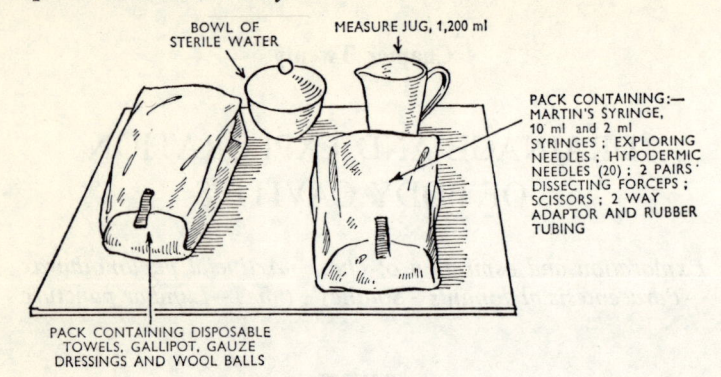

FIG. 106
Trolley for aspiration of chest. (See also Fig. 50.)

ARTIFICIAL PNEUMOTHORAX

This is the introduction of air into the pleural cavity in order to collapse the lung when it is necessary to rest a diseased part of that organ as in tuberculosis.

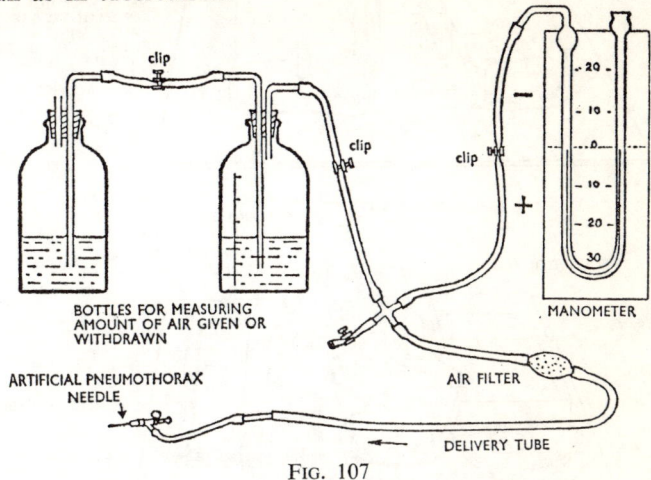

Fig. 107
Lillington Pearson apparatus for artificial pneumothorax.

Pneumoperitoneum

It may be useful to note here this procedure of introduction of air into the *peritoneal* cavity in order to collapse the lung when the apex of the lower lobe is involved, or when there is disease of both lungs, as a pre-operative measure.

PARACENTESIS ABDOMINIS

This is the procedure used for the relief of ascites which is the term used for increase in peritoneal fluid. It may be caused by:

1. Systemic venous back pressure, *e.g.* in heart failure.
2. Renal failure, when there is general oedema.
3. Abdominal malignant disease, *e.g.* carcinoma of any abdominal organ.
4. Chronic inflammation, *e.g.* tuberculosis.
5. Portal hypertension, *e.g.* cirrhosis of liver.
6. Chylous ascites, *e.g.* obstruction of lymphatic drainage from abdomen.
7. Nutritional oedema, *e.g.* vitamin B deficiency such as beri-beri.
8. Polyserositis, effusion of fluid from any serous membrane.

PRACTICAL NOTES ON NURSING PROCEDURES

Requirements on a trolley:

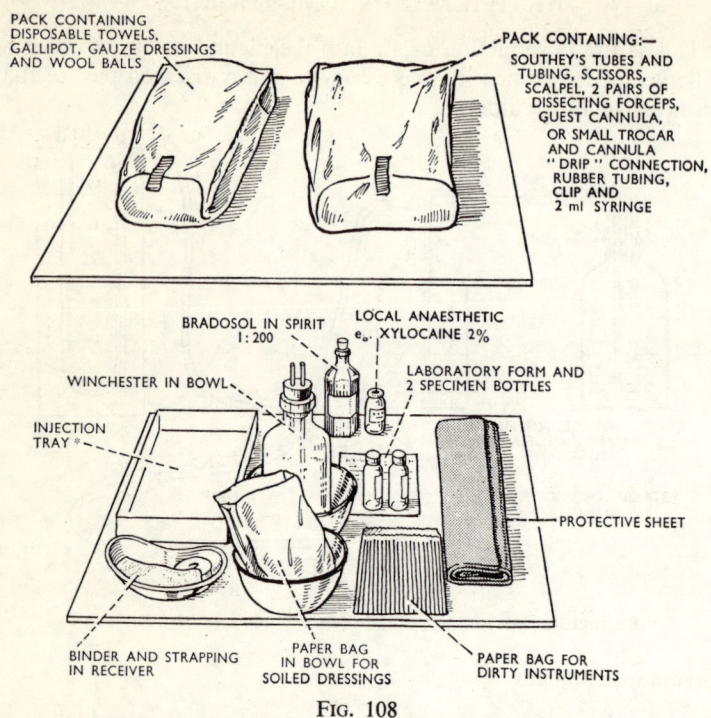

FIG. 108

Trolley for paracentesis abdominis. (See also Fig. 50.)

N.B.—Small plastic type cannulae with disposable metal introducers are now being produced.

Preparation of Patient:
1. Explain procedure to patient and screen bed.
2. Give bedpan or urinal.
3. Turn bedclothes down to top of thighs; cover chest with blanket.
4. Prop patient into sitting position.
5. Place binder behind patient in readiness. This may or may not be used, according to doctor's wishes.
6. During procedure watch pulse and adjust binder, if used, to maintain intra-abdominal pressure.
7. When completed or left to drain, make patient comfortable.
8. Clear away equipment. Measure fluid.

N.B.—When procedure is completed, cannula is removed and small patch dressing applied. Important to return trocar and cannula together with C.S.S.D.

SOUTHEY'S TUBES AND ACUPUNCTURE

These are two other methods used for relieving oedema.

1. *Southey's Tubes.*—Small cannulae are introduced into the subcutaneous tissue of the legs and thighs, rubber tubing attached and allowed to drain into dishes or thick pads of gamgee tissue.
2. *Acupuncture.*—Small incisions with a sharp scalpel are made into the skin of legs and thighs and allowed to drain into large pads of gamgee tissue.

For both procedures the patient should be sitting up in a chair if possible.

These two procedures are rarely used nowadays.

LUMBAR PUNCTURE

Requirements on a trolley:

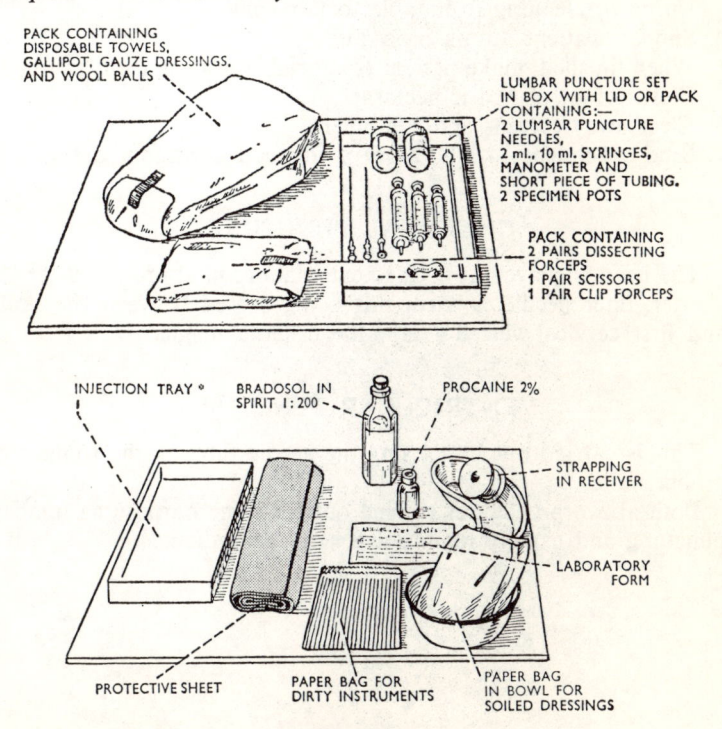

FIG. 109

Trolley for lumbar puncture. (See also Fig. 50.)

A lumbar puncture is carried out for the purpose of:
1. Obtaining a specimen of cerebro-spinal fluid for examination.
2. Relieving intra-cranial pressure, *e.g.* hydrocephaliis.
3. Administering drugs or anaesthetics.

Bed elevator in readiness under the bed.
Stool or chair required for doctor.

Preparation of the patient:

1. Explain procedure to patient if possible and screen bed. Give bedpan or urinal.
2. Place trolley in position, remove all but one pillow and turn bedclothes down to pubes. Cover patient with small blanket. If male patient and area hairy, this may need shaving.
3. Position of patient. May be (*a*) *left lateral* with spine well flexed, head down on chest and knees drawn up to abdomen or (*b*) *sitting up*, leaning over table to flex spine.
4. Support patient during procedure.
5. When finished, make patient comfortable in recumbent position. Elevate foot of bed if necessary.
6. Clear away screens and equipment.
7. Send specimens to laboratory if instructed, without delay.

CISTERNAL PUNCTURE

The head is shaved at back to external occipital protuberance. A shorter, finer needle is used, this being passed between the skull and first cervical vertebra into the cisterna magna.

VENTRICULAR PUNCTURE

This is carried out by passing the needle through the fontanelle or burr-holes.

Both above procedures carried out for same purpose as lumbar puncture, and usually require a general anaesthetic.

Chapter Twenty-one

LABORATORY EXAMINATIONS

Urine concentration, urea clearance and concentration tests—Blood tests—Cerebro-spinal fluid—Sternal puncture—Fractional test meal—Histamine test—Glucose tolerance test

Water excretion and urine concentration test

There is no special preparation of the patient.

5.0 p.m.	Give 1 pint of fluid (water, tea or coffee) with a meal. No further food or fluid is allowed until the test is completed.
7.0 p.m. to 7.0 a.m.	Empty bladder and discard urine.
7.0 p.m.	Collect all urine in one bottle and label 'Night'.
8.0 a.m.	Collect all urine; label 1.
9.0 a.m.	Collect all urine; label 2.
10.0 a.m.	Collect all urine; label 3.
11.0 a.m.	Collect all urine; label 4.

Urea clearance test, for excretory efficiency of kidneys

Normal: 70 to 80 per cent.

There is no special preparation of the patient except that tea or coffee should be taken early, before breakfast.

SPECIMENS REQUIRED:

1. Initial urine at a noted time.
2. All the urine for next one-hour period.
3. All the urine for next (second) one-hour period.

To facilitate collection of hourly urine samples, a half-pint of water should be given to patient at the beginning of each hour.

A blood sample should also be collected from the vein in an Oxalate bottle at about end of first hour of test period.

Urea concentration test

Normal: 2 to 3 per cent.

Patient is allowed nothing to eat or drink for twelve hours preceding test; *i.e.* after 8.0 p.m. previous night. Following specimens are required:

1. Urine specimen to empty bladder completely at a noted time (say 9.0 a.m.).
   A dose of urea is then given immediately by mouth.
2. All urine for one hour following the dose.
3. All urine for next (second) hour.
4. All urine for next (third) hour.

For adults dose is:
Urea	15 grammes.
Tincture of orange	1 ml.
Water	Up to 100 ml.

For children the dose of urea is proportioned to age as follows:

Age in years	*Grammes of urea*
8 to 12	12
5 to 8	10
3 to 5	7
1 to 3	6
Under 1	4

Urea range test

Patient should have ordinary diet but minimum of fluids from mid-day onwards.

9.0 p.m.	Patient is given 15 grammes urea in 4 oz water.
10.0 p.m.	Urine is obtained and discarded.
10.0 p.m. to 6.0. a.m.	All urine is collected as specimen A.
6.0 a.m.	Patient is given 30 oz water or weak tea.
7.0 a.m. to 12 noon.	Urine is collected *every hour*, *i.e.* six separate complete specimens are obtained and sent to the laboratory together with specimen A (above).

Blood count

Normal: Hb 85 to 105 per cent.
Red cells 5,000,000 per c.mm.
White cells 6,000 to 8,000 per c.mm.
Platelets 250,000 per c.mm.

LABORATORY EXAMINATIONS

Blood urea
Normal: 20 to 40 mg per 100 ml.

Blood sugar
Normal: 80 to 120 mg per 100 ml (fasting); after meals 180.

Blood sedimentation rate (ESR)
Westergren: 1 to 8 mm in one hour.

Blood clotting
Normal: 3 to 4 minutes.
Prothrombin time: 10 to 14 seconds.

Wassermann and Kahn
Specimens for all blood tests taken by laboratory staff, for diagnosis of syphilis.

Occult blood, not visible to the naked eye
Three days before, no foods containing haemoglobin derivatives are given, *i.e.* no meat or fish, no iron medicines, green vegetables or purgatives of vegetable origin.
Collect specimen of stool in special container.

Hippuric acid synthesis test, for efficiency of liver functon
Patient is given a light breakfast. One hour later urine is discarded and the test begun. A dose of 6 grammes sodium benzoate dissolved in 1 or 2 oz of water and flavoured with oil of peppermint is given to patient; followed by half a glass of water. *All* urine for the next period of 4 hours is collected for analysis.

Liver and kidney biopsy
Carried out by doctor using a special needle to obtain specimen of liver or kidney substance.

Jejunum biopsy
Taken with Crosbie capsule, for diagnosing steatorrhoea. Crosbie

capsule—a long fine plastic tube with a metal capsule on the end. The patient has the tube passed and is then screened in the X-ray department. When the capsule is in the jejunum, the tube is aspirated causing the capsule to 'bite off' a piece of jejunal mucosa. The tube is then carefully withdrawn and specimen removed.

Xylase test

To estimate enzyme deficiency or bowel wall dysfunction.
6 a.m. patient empties bladder, urine is discarded.
    Xylase powder 25 mg given with two tumblers of water to drink.
7 a.m. one tumbler of water given.
8 a.m. one tumbler of water given.

All urine passed from 6 a.m. until 11 a.m. is saved and sent to laboratory.

Cerebro-spinal fluid

Normal:
Pressure	60 to 150 mm.
Cells	0 to 5 lymphocytes per c.mm.
Chlorides	700 to 760 mg/100 ml.
Glucose	70 to 100 mg/100 ml.
Protein	10 to 35 mg/100 ml.
Urea	10 to 40 mg/100 ml.

Sternal puncture

To obtain a specimen of bone marrow.

Requirements on a trolley:

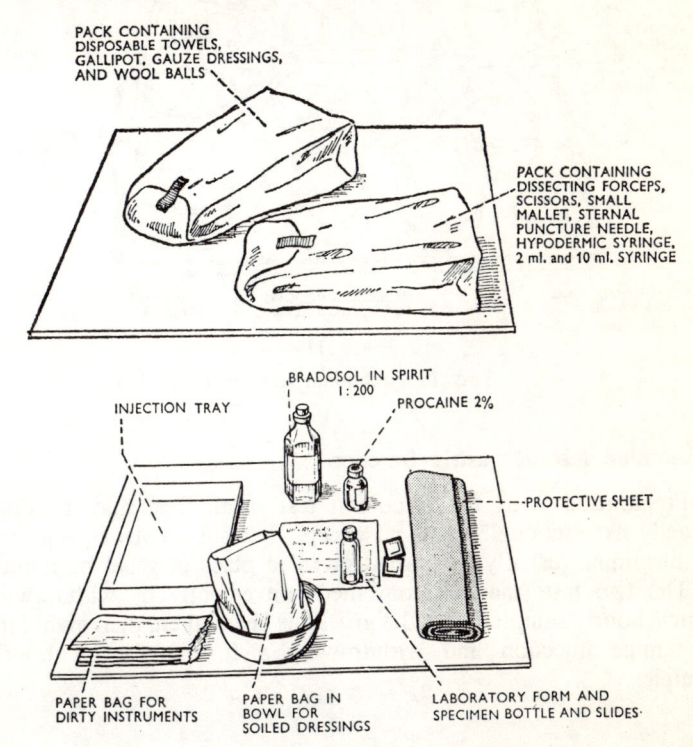

FIG. 110
Trolley for sternal puncture. (See also Fig. 50.)

Small area on man's chest may require shaving.

Fractional test meal

To estimate amount of hydrochloric acid in gastric juice.

Patient should take two charcoal biscuits with light meal on evening preceding test. Nothing further to eat or drink is permitted. After at least 12 hours fasting, stomach contents are removed completely. Gruel (salt free but may be sweetened) is then given and samples of gastric contents obtained $\frac{1}{4}$ hourly for 2 hours.

Gruel test meal rarely used nowadays.

194 PRACTICAL NOTES ON NURSING PROCEDURES

Requirements on a tray:

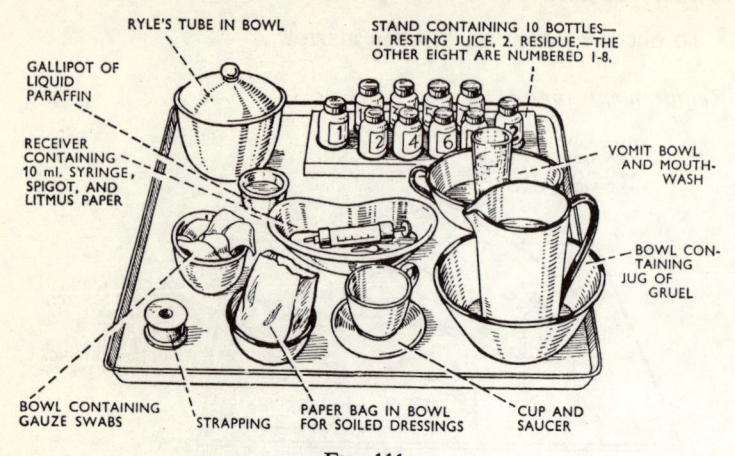

Fig. 111
Tray for fractional test meal.

Histamine test of gastric function

Preparation is as for fractional test meal. Test may be done exactly as fractional test meal except that subcutaneous injection of histamine (usually 0·5 mg) is given in place of gruel by mouth.

The two tests may be combined conveniently by withdrawing four $\frac{1}{4}$ hourly samples after the gruel has been taken, then giving the histamine injection and withdrawing a further four $\frac{1}{4}$ hourly samples.

Quinine test meal

1. Patient drinks 1 pint of bland fluid the night before (9 p.m.).
2. Breakfast to be omitted.
3. (*a*) Empty bladder (8 a.m.). *This sample to be discarded.*
   (*b*) Immediately after swallow capsule supplied in $\frac{1}{2}$ glass of water. If difficulty is experienced in swallowing it, empty it into water and wash down with further $\frac{1}{2}$ glass of water. Capsule contains 250 mg of caffeine-sodium-benzoate to act as a diuretic.
4. Wait 1 hour (9 a.m.). Pass *Control urine.* Retain in appropriately labelled bottle. Then immediately afterwards (*a*) drink suspension of *quinine resin* in $\frac{1}{2}$ glass of water. Do not chew. Wash down with a further $\frac{1}{2}$ glass of water. (*b*) Give injection of histamine (0·5 mg) S/C.
5. After 1 hour (10 a.m.) pass urine sample No. 1. Keep.

6. After 2 hours (11 a.m.) pass urine sample No. 2. Keep. Put in appropriate bottles. Test completed.

Notes:

1. No restrictions are placed on smoking, exercise, etc., and test can begin at any hour.
2. Medication with iron, aluminium, magnesium preparations, and vitamins should be withheld for 48 hours prior to test.

Glucose tolerance test, for liver function

Patient has no food for 12 hours preceding test, *i.e.* 9 p.m. previous night, except that a little water or tea without sugar may be given at 7 a.m. A sample of venous blood is collected in a fluoride bottle and a sample of urine is also obtained. The patient is then given a test dose of glucose, 0·5 g per pound body-weight (but not exceeding 100 g glucose). For most adults, a test of 50 g glucose dissolved in a tumbler of water is usual without specific reference to the body weight. Further blood samples are collected in fluoride bottles at $\frac{1}{2}$-hourly intervals, after the dose of glucose, up to $2\frac{1}{2}$-hour point, and a further specimen of urine is collected covering the $2\frac{1}{2}$-hour test period.

Shows ability of liver to convert glucose to glycogen, measuring approximate severity of diabetes mellitus.

Galactose and laevulose tolerance tests, for liver function

Patient has no food for 12 hours preceding test, *i.e.* after 9 p.m. previous night, except that a little water or tea without sugar may be given at 7 a.m.

(*a*) Elimination of more than 3 g of galactose over a 5-hour period indicates liver dysfunction.

(*b*) Blood sugar level normally unaffected by oral administration of laevulose—increased in presence of liver disease.

Base metabolic rate

Patient is allowed no food at all after 9 p.m. previous night. Essential requirement is to secure complete physical and mental relaxation in the morning at time of test. To induce this relaxation, patient's comfort should be ensured by sponging hands and face, attention to bowels and bladder and avoidance of undue thirst by mouth-wash or giving a little water to drink, early in morning.

Height, weight and age of patient are all required for calculation of B.M.R. and should be noted previously; send note with patient at time of test. Patient's temperature should be normal, so check beforehand.

Normal +10 to −10 per cent.

Chapter Twenty-two

ANAESTHETICS.
ARTIFICIAL RESPIRATORS

Preparation for anaesthetics—Hypothermia—Types of respirators —Care of patient

ANAESTHETIC

Anaesthetic trolley for inhalant and intravenous anaesthetics

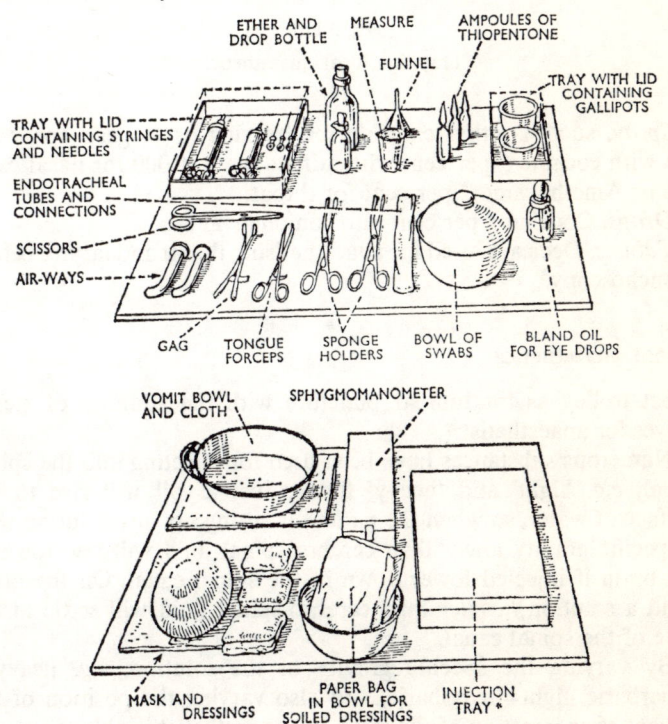

FIG. 112

Trolley for inhalant and intravenous anaesthetics. (See also Fig. 50.)

Rectal. Tray as for intermittent rectal saline. Pentothal.
Oral. E.g. Nembutal or sodium amytal.

Tray for local anaesthetic

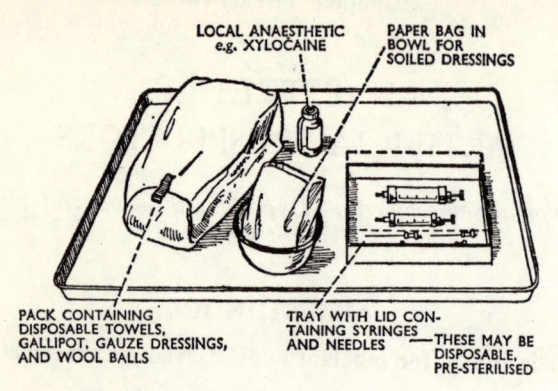

FIG. 113
Tray for local anaesthetic.

Spray, such as ethyl chloride for freezing or Roger's spray for use with cocaine 5 per cent with adrenaline 1 : 1,000 for nasal cavities or Amethocaine 2 per cent for throat.

Drops. Cocaine 2 per cent into conjunctival sac.

Tablets. Decicain, used for anaesthetising throat and larynx before bronchoscopy.

Spinal anaesthetics

Set trolley as for lumbar puncture with the addition of sterile gloves for anaesthetist.

Numerous substances have been used for injecting into the spinal canal, *e.g.* 'light' and 'heavy' fluids. Just as oil will rise to the surface of water, so when the patient is sitting up, any solution with a specific gravity *lower* than cerebro-spinal fluid will rise towards the brain if injected lower down in the spinal canal. On the other hand a solution *heavier* than cerebro-spinal fluid will settle at the base of the spinal canal.

By varying the specific gravity of the solution, *e.g.* heavy= hyperbaric, light=hypobaric, and also varying the position of the patient after injection of the fluid, the anaesthetist is able to control the level of the spinal cord at which the drug will work. Because of this, spinal anaesthetics are described as 'high spinal' and 'low spinal'. The higher the level, the greater will be the degree of blood vessel paralysis and the greater therefore, will be the risk of low blood pressure and shock.

ANAESTHETICS. ARTIFICIAL RESPIRATORS

When the patient returns to the ward after a spinal anaesthetic, whatever the type used, he should be placed flat in bed for 24 hours unless instructions are given to the contrary.

Hypothermia

The cooling of a patient to a temperature of 30° C (86° F) for the purpose of carrying out *surgical operations*, *e.g.* valvular lesions of the heart.

The lowering of the temperature to 30° C reduces the oxygen consumption of the brain by two thirds, this allows occlusion of circulation for 8 to 10 minutes without brain damage.

Surface cooling is carried out by wrapping patient in ice cold blankets and packing round with icebags, or immersion in ice cold water.

Systemic cooling can be achieved by bleeding patient from an artery, the blood being passed through a long length of rubber tubing which is immersed in ice cold water, and then being returned to patient's vein.

Another method is by use of Largactil which as well as acting on the temperature regulating mechanism of the body and preventing patient from shivering, also reduces metabolism. Largactil together with phenergan appears to depress the human body to a state of artificial hibernation.

Very important to avoid prolonged or severe pressure on any part of the body during hypothermia.

Post-operative nursing care requires most careful supervision.

ARTIFICIAL RESPIRATORS

Types

1. Tank or cabinet respirator, *e.g.* Modified Both. Drinker.
2. Cuirass, *e.g.* Kifa. Monaghan.
3. Bragg Paul, *e.g.* inflatable pneumatic jacket.
4. The rocking bed.
   These are all negative pressure type respirators.
5. Beaver pneumoflator.
6. Oxford inflator.
   Both positive pressure respirators.

To place patient in cabinet respirator

With the negative pressure control valve being at 8, the motor is started and the platform is made up ready for the patient with a sheet, plastic and cotton draw sheets. A top sheet and one or two blankets are placed in readiness. A rubber bedpan may be placed in position if necessary. The patient is dressed in an open-backed flannel gown and woollen stockings. A collar of lint greased with petroleum jelly, is placed round his neck and lightly bandaged in position. He is then lifted by at least three people on to the prepared platform with his neck resting comfortably in lower neckpiece. Shoulder pads are placed in position to prevent pressure. The foot-piece is adjusted for comfort and the patient covered with sheet and blankets. After the platform has been pushed into the cabinet and fastened the upper neck-piece is put on and the upper portion of the front is then closed and fastened. The neck-piece should fit comfortably and not too tightly, cotton wool being used to seal off any air-leaks between collar and patient's neck.

The head rest is carefully adjusted. Care must be taken to see that the machine is level and the legs firmly fixed before the platform is pushed in, also that there is no obstruction to prevent proper closing of the cabinet, *e.g.* bedclothes, after the platform is pushed in.

The negative pressure is then adjusted to 16 to 18 cm of water either by a dial manometer or a water manometer. The rate of respiration depends on the physician's orders.

When the respirator is working satisfactorily and the patient's airway is free from obstruction, *e.g.* mucus removed by a sucker, the patient will:

1. Rest comfortably and improve in colour.
2. Stop breathing voluntarily. The respiratory movements will synchronise with the respirator.
3. Lose anxiety and fear and will probably fall asleep.

Nursing care

The patient must not be left unattended.

There may be pyrexia and pain and tenderness of muscles during the first day or two and there may be general discomfort.

If there is no movement of respiratory muscles the patient must receive nursing care through the port-holes. In most cases it is possible to open the cabinet for a short period especially if there is a positive pressure apparatus available.

Care of the skin and all pressure areas is important, so that, if possible, a daily blanket bath should be given and treatment for the prevention of pressure sores conscientiously carried out together with the frequent change of position and protection of bony prominences by small rings, pads and pillows.

The skin of the neck requires particular care to prevent sores developing from the friction of the collar.

The mouth and teeth must receive regular attention to keep them clean and moist.

The hair should be done in the most comfortable way, *e.g.* two plaits tied with tape if long.

Adequate fluids must be administered in the form of small sips of water or fruit juices, care being taken that aspiration of fluids into the lungs does not occur. An angular glass tube is a convenient means of giving drinks and the patient soon learns to adjust his swallowing to the rhythm of the bellows.

After the acute stage the diet is gradually increased until the patient is taking a full diet.

To relieve constipation, small enemas or glycerine suppositories may be given on alternate days, but where there is paralysis of the abdominal muscles and of the gut these may be retained. Under these circumstances it may be necessary to give Pitressin or, as a last resort, manual removal of faeces may be necessary.

Retention of urine must be reported and dealt with as ordered, but if catheterisation is necessary, strict asepsis must be used.

ORTHOPAEDIC TREATMENT.—This is ordered by the surgeon and carried out by the physiotherapist, but maintenance of good positions depends on adequate nursing supervision.

PSYCHOLOGICAL TREATMENT.—Constant reassurance, kindness and encouragement are necessary to allay fears of the patient. Gentleness and sympathy together with firmness and quiet are also necessary. There must be no discussion of the patient within his hearing. Mirrors may be fitted so that the patient can see a little of what is going on.

When the patient is removed from the cabinet for nursing treatment the motor should not be stopped.

When the patient has recovered the full use of the respiratory muscles he should be taken out of the respirator gradually, *e.g.* for 20 minutes, then 1 hour, increasing the length of time until he can be out altogether.

It is advisable in the early stages to leave the motor on while he is out.

Tracheostomy is now frequently performed to be used in conjunction with artificial respirators, particularly those of the positive pressure type.

APPENDIX

Mouth feeding in special cases

HARELIP AND CLEFT PALATE.—Special spoons can be obtained for feeding babies with harelips who are unable to suck.

Teats with a flange to fit over the hard palate can be used for babies with cleft palates.

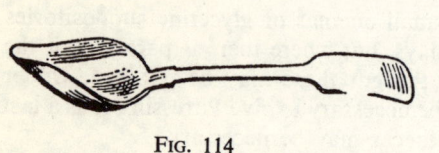

FIG. 115
Flanged teat for babies with cleft palate.

FIG. 114
Special spoon for babies with harelips.

TONGUE OPERATIONS AND JAW INJURIES.—A feeding cup with a piece of rubber tubing attached to the spout is usually the easiest method of feeding these cases. It is most important to keep spout and rubber tubing scrupulously clean.

Feeds should always be followed by sterile water to help keep the patient's mouth clean.

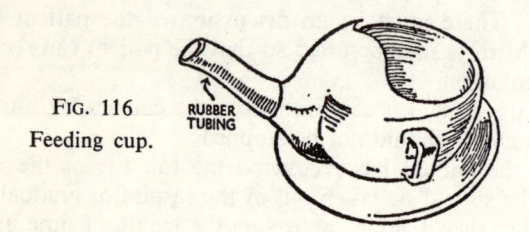

FIG. 116
Feeding cup.

Intubation

Consists of introducing a tube into the larynx through the mouth. The tube has a piece of silk thread attached with which to fasten it to the face in front of the ear by a small piece of adhesive strapping.

Used occasionally in obstruction of the larynx.

High colonic irrigation

Fluid in fairly large quantities, *e.g.* normal saline or plain water, 8 pints, is injected into the rectum and colon, 2 pints at a time, and then syphoned back, or patient is allowed to evacuate bowel into suitable receptacle.

It is a drastic treatment and careful watch must be kept on patient's general condition.

Underwater or closed drainage

This is achieved by the tube from the patient being connected to a glass tube which passes through the bung of the drainage bottle, into a known quantity of sterile water or antiseptic, preventing air returning up the tube. There is also a thistle funnel placed in the bung, filled with cotton wool to act as a filter, at the same time allowing air to enter bottle.

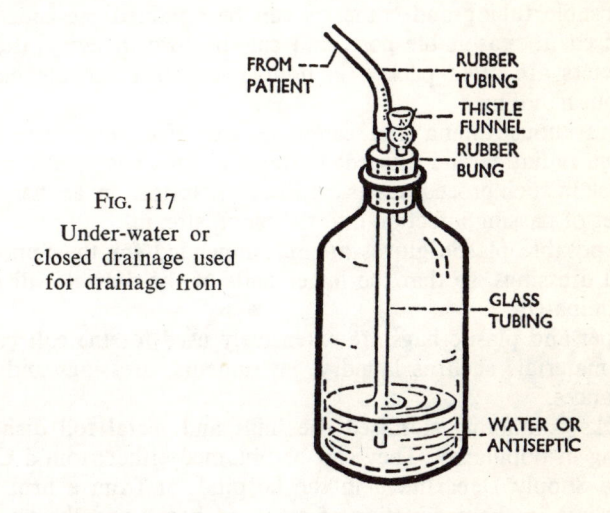

FIG. 117
Under-water or closed drainage used for drainage from

Electro-convulsive therapy

This is carried out for the treatment of depressive states. The patient is given a general anaesthetic, *e.g.* pentothal and also a muscle relaxant, after which an electric current is passed through the head sufficient to produce a modified convulsion. Oxygen must be available.

Some disposable items which are now available:

Catheters—Female
        Foley
        Gibbons
        Harris

Masks
Medi-plast bag and tubing
    for drainage
Nylon film for packs

St. Peter's	Oxygen mask
Whistle tip	Polythene mattress covers
Dishes and gallipots—tinfoil	Surgeon's caps
Finger stalls	Syringes and needles
Gloves	Towels
Intracath cannula	Translet colostomy set
Intravenous cannula	Trays—cardboard
Intravenous recipient set	

Disposable items are being more widely used as their value in preventing cross infection in hospitals, clinics, surgeries, and factories, is realised.

Rubber tubing and catheters are extremely difficult to clean properly after they have been used for draining body cavities. Disposable tubing and catheters can be obtained pre-packed and sterilised at reasonable cost, and can be thrown away after use. Catheters are often packed in double jackets to enable insertion without handling.

Intravenous tubing and cannulae are effectively sterilised by gamma radiation and discarded after use. This has greatly reduced the risk in such procedures as cardiac catheterisation, as there is less danger of passing infection into the blood stream.

Disposable plastic gloves are recommended for the removal of soiled dressings, so that the finger nails of the dresser will not be contaminated.

Paper and plastic bags are extensively used for the collection of used materials such as laundry, instruments, dressings and waste substances.

Packs containing sterilised dressings and metal foil dishes are gaining in popularity. They can be obtained either from a Central Sterile Supply Department in the hospital, or from a firm which specialises in the production of standard packs and the necessary accessories. These save a great deal of nursing staff time, and when the correct way of using them has been learned, reduce the possibility of spread of infection.

Disposable enema apparatus saves time, and is less uncomfortable for the patient.

Disposable colostomy bags which are conveniently emptied and then discarded, are very helpful.

Paper towels, babies' napkins, pads for the incontinent, sheets for out-patient couches, and even caps and gowns for nurses, obviously save laundry bills and linen replacements, but their bulk when used in large numbers, creates difficulty in disposal, especially in smokeless zones.

Disposable bedpans have been tried, but require a special machine for crushing, and apparently some local sewage disposal units cannot deal with the waste material produced. The storage of large numbers can also be a problem.

On the whole disposable items can be of great benefit. They assist in bringing about improved standards of hygiene. Nursing staff time can be saved and the work made easier. Laundry costs and linen replacements can be reduced, and sterilisers may become redundant. Patients are less embarrassed by hidden polythene bags collecting urine, than by glass containers on the floor. On the other hand disposable items are so easy to use that they may be wastefully employed and in this direction hospital costs are soaring. Paper towels or napkins are not necessarily best for the human skin. Common sense is needed as much in the use of disposables, as in all other things. Disposable syringes and needles should be safely discarded, *i.e.* the needle junction should be broken off, rendering the syringe unusable. Pressurised containers when empty must not be put in the incinerator or they will explode.

Illustrations of disposable articles appear frequently in the Nursing Press.

INDEX

INDEX

INDEX

Acupuncture, 187
Admission, emergency, 48
  observations by nurse, 48
  procedure, 47
Aerated bath, 135
Aerosol therapy, 106
Ambulant patient, 66
Ammonia, 105
Amyl nitrate, 105
Anaesthetics, inhalant, 197
  intravenous, 197
  local, 198
  spinal, 198
Antiphlogistine, 132
Antiseptic bath, 135
Antrostomy, 168
Antrum washout, 168
Aortography, 123
Apnoea, 70
Artificial feeding, gastrostomy, 173
  jejunostomy, 174
  nasal and oesophageal, 174, 175
Artificial pneumothorax, 185
Artificial respirators, nursing care of patients in, 200, 201
  placing patients in, 199
  types of, 199
Asphyxia, 70
Auricular fibrillation, 69
Auscultation, 121
Autoclave, 91

Barium meal and enema, 122
Basal metabolic rate, 195
Bathing, children, 53
  infants, 53, 54, 55
Baths, temperature, 135
  varieties, 135
Bed accessories, air bed, 43
  air-rings, 42
  bedpans, 45
  bedrests, 42
  cradles, 42
  elevators, 42
  fracture boards, 43
  hot water bottles, 43
  locker, 44
  pulleys, 44
  ripple bed, 43
  sandbags, 41
  stripper, 31
  urinals, 45

Bed bathing, 52, 53
Bedmaking, changing bottom sheet, 31
  empty bed, 29, 30
  general rules, 29
  occupied bed, 30
Bedpans, to clean, 22
  giving and removing, 64
  washers, to clean, 22
Bedsores, causes of, 56
  frequency of treatment, 57
  method of treatment, 57, 58
  pressure areas, 56
  routine preventive treatment, 56
  types of patients liable to, 56
Bedstead, 26
Bladder washout, female, 149
  male, 149, 150
Blankets, 27
  washing and sterilising, 28
B.L.B. (Boothby, Lovelace, Bulbulian) masks, 108
Blood, clotting, 191
  count, 190
  donors, 181
  prothrombin time, 191
  sedimentation, 191
  sugar, 191
  urea, 191
Blood pressure, taking and recording, 71, 72, 73
Bradycardia, 69
Breakdown in health, factors contributing to, 17
British College of Nurses, 8
Bronchoscopy, 127

Carbon dioxide, administration of, 109
Cardiac beds, acute and chronic, 33
Cardiac catheterisation, 123
Catheterisation, female, 145, 146
  male, 147
Central Sterile Supply Department, 93
Cerebro-spinal fluid, 192
Chest, aspiration of, 183, 184
  exploration of, 183
Cheyne-Stokes' respiration, 70
Cholecystography, 122
Cisternal puncture, 188

Cleaning, electric lights, 21
  floors, 21
  glass, 21
  kitchen, 21
  lavatory and sluice, 22
  metal, 21
  screen and trolley wheels, 21
  sterilising room, 22
  walls, 21
  ward bathroom, 22
  woodwork, 21
Cleft palate, 202
Cold compress, 129
Colostomy washout, 152
Commodes, 65
Cot making, 32
Counter-irritants, 134
Cystoscopy, 126

Departments of the hospital, 1
Dilatation and curettage, 127
Dilution of, lotions, 97
  potent drugs, 97
Discharge, 48
Disinfectants, 92
Disinfection, 91
Disposable items, 203, 204
Divided bed, 36, 37
Dyspnoea, 70

Ear, instillation of drops, 163
  syringing, 162
Electric thermometers, 69
Electro-convulsive therapy, 203
Emergency admission beds, 32
Emollient bath, 135
Enema saponis, 83
Enemata, complications, 83
  reasons for use, 81
  requirements and method, 82
Equipment for beds, 25
Ethics, 8
Etiquette, 8
Ethylene oxide, 91
Evaporating compress, 130
Excretion urography, 122
Extra systole, 69
Extravasation of urine, 76
Extensions, 138, 139
Eye, instillation of drops, 170
  irrigation, 171, 172
  spoon bathing and swabbing, 171

Faeces, abnormal characteristics, 76
  consistency, 76
  substances in, 77
  normal, 76
  specimens, 77

Feet, care of, 61
Fever, continuous, 68
  intermittent, 68
  remittent, 68
Fluid measurement, 86, 87
Foam bath, 135
Fomentation, surgical, 131
Fractional test meal, 193, 194
Fracture bed, 35

Galactose tolerance test, 195
Gamma irradiation, 91
Gastric aspiration, continuous, 161
  intermittent, 159
Gastroscopy, 127
General nursing care, 116
General Nursing Council, 5, 6
General observation of patients, 114
Getting patient up, 65
Gifts, 9
Glucose tolerance test, 195
Glycerine suppositories, 83

Hands, care of, 60
Harelip, 202
Head and hair, care of, 61
  indications for inspection, 62
  washing in bed, 62, 63, 64
Health, nurses' influence in teaching, 16, 17
  teaching of, 16
Heating, 19
High colonic irrigation, 202
Hippuric acid synthesis test, 191
Histamine test, 194
Hospital, economy, 23, 24, 25
  functions of, 1
  points to remember in, 12, 13
  routine, 2
Hot water bottles, care and use of, 46
Hyperpnoea, 70
Hypertonic saline, enema, 84
Hypodermic injections, 100
Hypothermia, 199
Hypoxaemia, 107

Icebag, 130
Incontinence of urine, 75
Infant feeding, 55
Infection, measures to prevent spread, 88
  sources of, 88
  spread of, 88
Influence of environment in illness, 15
Infusions, bone marrow, 181
  intravenous, 179, 180, 181
  subcutaneous, 177, 178

INDEX

Inhalations, dry, 105
  Nelson's inhaler, 103
  steam tent or canopy, 104, 105
International Council of Nurses, 18
Intramuscular injections, 101
Intubation, 168, 202
Isolation nursing, 89

Jaw injuries, feeding in, 202
Jejunum biopsy, 191

Kahn test, 191
Kaolin poultice, 132

Laevulose tolerance test, 195
Laryngoscopy, 127
Last offices, 49, 50, 51
Legal aspects, 12
Lighting, 19
Linen, care of, 28
  to disinfect, 27
  to prepare for laundry, 28
  varieties, 27
Liniments, 134
Liver and kidney biopsy, 191
Lumbar puncture, 187, 188

Magnesium sulphate enema, 83
Mattress frame, 26
Mattresses, 26, 27
Medicines, administration of, 98
  alternative methods of giving, 99
  rules for giving, 98
  storage, 97
Micturition, 74
Ministry of Health and Social Security, 3
Mouth and teeth, care of, 59
  dentures, 59
  reason for treatment, 60
  result of neglect, 60
Myringotomy, requirements for, 168

Nasal bleeding, control of, 169
Nasal washout, 164
Nobecutane spray, 94
Noise in hospital, 19
Normal saline enema, 84
Nose, cleaning, 164
  instillation of drops, 164
Nurses' Act, 4

Occult blood, 191
Oesophagoscopy, 126
Ointments, 134
Olive oil enema, 83
Orthopnoea, 70
Out-patients, 3
Oxygen, general management, 106
  nasal, 107
  tents, 108

Palpation, 121
Paracentesis abdominis, 185, 186
Patients' wills, 12
Percentage solutions, 96
Percussion, 121
Peritoneoscopy, 127
Peritonsillar abscess, requirements for opening, 169
Physical examinations, abdomen, 118
  chest, 118
  ear and eye, 117
  general, 121
  nervous system, 121
  nose and throat, 118
  rectum, 119
  vagina, 120
Pillows, 27
Plaster bed, dry, 35
  wet, 36
Plaster of Paris, anterior shells, 142
  applications of, 140
  bandages, 140
  beds, 142
  casts, 142
  drying of, 141
  requirements for, 140
  slabs, 142
  tightness of, 141
Pneumoperitoneum, 185
Positions, dorsal, 39
  genu-pectoral, 40
  left lateral, 40
  lithotomy, 40
  prone, 38
  recumbent, 37
  semi-recumbent, 38
  Sim's, 40
  Trendelenburg, 41
  upright, 39
Post-anaesthetic tray, 35
Post-operation bed, 34
Post-operative care, 113
Post-operative observations, 113
Pre-operative treatment, 110
Pre-operative shaving, 112
Psychological aspect of nursing, 13, 14
Pulse, 69
  taking and recording, 71
Pyrexia, termination of, 68
  types of, 68

Quantitative test for chlorides, 81
Quinine test, 194

Radio-active isotopes, 125
Radio-active tracers, 125
Radium therapy, 123
Rectal tube, 84
Rectal washout, 151

Relationship, between nurse and patient, 14
  between nurse and relatives, 15
Removal of, excreta from floors, 23
  stains from linen, blood, 22
    ink, 22
    tea, coffee, cocoa, 22
    fruit, 23
    rust marks, 23
Reports, writing, 116
Respiration, taking and recording, 71
  types of, 70
Responsibilities of nurse to patient, 15
Retention enema, 85
Retention of urine, 75
  causes and treatment, 75
Rigor, 68
Routine, 20
Royal British Nurses' Association, 7
Royal College of Nursing, 7

Sanichairs, 65
Scott's dressing, 134
Shallow respiration, 70
Sighing, 70
Sigmoidoscopy, 126
Silicone Vasogen, 57
Simple enema, 83
Sinus arrhythmia, 69
Skin preparation, 113
Southey's tubes, 187
Splints, external, 142
  internal, 143
  padding, 143
Sponging, tepid, 136
Sputum, mugs, to clean, 22
  observations, 78
  precautions, 78
Starch poultice, 133
State Enrolled Nurse Regulations, 8
Sterilisation, 90, 91
Sternal puncture, 193
Stertorous breathing, 70
Stimulating bath, 135
Stomach washout, 158
Stramonium, 106
Stress incontinence, 75
Stridor, 70
Student Nurses' Association, 7
Suppression of urine, 75

Tachycardia, 69
Tampons, 156

Temperature, inverse, 67
  taking and recording, 70
Test for, acetone, 80
  albumen, 79
  bile, 80
  blood, 80
  diacetic acid, 80
  pus, 80
  sugar, 80
Thoracoscopy, 127
Throat, gargling, 165
  painting, 165
  spraying, 165
Tidal drainage, 150
Tongue operations, feeding after, 202
Tracheotomy, after care, 166, 167
  requirements, 166
Traction, indications, 138
  nursing points, 138, 139
  requirements, 139
  types, 138
Turkish bath, 135

Unconscious patient, 114, 115
Under-water drainage bottle, 203
Unna's paste, 134
Urea, clearance test, 189
  concentration test, 189, 190
  range test, 190
Urinals, to clean, 22
Urine, composition, 74
  concentration test, 189
  specimens, 76
  testing, 79

Vaginal douching, 154
Vaginal irrigation, 155
Vaginal pessaries, 156
Vapour baths, 135
Ventilation, 19
Ventricular puncture, 188
Vomit, observations of, 79
  contents of, 79, 80, 81

Ward dressing technique, 93
Wassermann test, 191
Weights and measures, approximate equivalents, 95, 96
  domestic measures, 96
  imperial, 95
  metric, 95
Wheezing, 70
Whitley Council, 6, 7

X-ray examinations, 122
Xylase test, 192